Bulletproof Your Immune System

Preface

It's an indisputable fact that we are in our best health in our younger years, but that doesn't mean you can't or shouldn't be when you're older. It doesn't just happen. In fact there's a tried and true strategy based on science, principles, physiology, and first-hand experience that can and will repair, restore, and build your immune system to be virtually bulletproof, at any age.

One thing that is telling comes by way of the medical community when they admit they don't know why an elderly person who has the health profile of a young healthy individual poses a greater risk for disease, virus, and depression. It's that revelation that tells me they're not considering how important it is to address the unbelievable power and strength of physiology. When you build physiological and emotional strength, you've now created a foundation and natural barrier for fighting and eliminating all diseases, end of story.

The key to success is the manipulation of critical components responsible for weaponizing your emotional and physical state of being. They are so important that even leaving one of them out of the equation compromises overall results. However, when they are implemented together, your mind and body become bulletproof to disease, viruses, and depression.

The truth is, the medical community has made some remarkable breakthroughs in medicine, but I'm stunned by what they don't know, as in the example of not knowing why healthy, older individuals are automatically more exposed to disease. I don't buy it, in fact I think some doctors have their heads in the sand. I believe it's because of the lack of first-hand experience, in addition to discounting the true power of mind and body.

This book will reveal a step-by-step process on how to fortify overall health, based on my own 38 years of experience, and backed by physical evidence from my personal up to date lab work showing the profile of an 18-year-old healthy male. Considering I'm 65 years of age, I would say the proof is in the pudding.

Part of the problem in our society is that we have a severe case of sheep mentality, which creates an environment of mediocrity, weakness, and being codependent on others.

If you aren't willing to think for yourself, you must be willing to accept the dire consequences. Enjoy your journey to the development of a bulletproof immune system, where you'll never again fear disease.

-Leo

Part One (Fill In)

Defeat Disease, Virus and Depression

State the objective

In order to get targeted results, you must shorten the learning curve by taking a direct approach, otherwise results will always be compromised. This strategy requires being very specific about the results you desire.

They recommendation is to list the top three priorities for your health and well being. Don't over think this process, just list your priorities in life based on what comes to mind.

You'll be surprised how powerful your intuition is, and your tendency toward a particular behavior that you may or may not want to work on. This is part of your hardwire, known as instinct. You have to trust that inner voice even though at times it may seem counterintuitive. The best thing to do in these scenarios is stay out of your own way and let your intuition and instinct guide you, because most of the time it will be right.

Goal 1:

____

____

Goal 2:

____

____

Goal 3:

____

____

These are the 3 goals we are going to focus on in the specific order you wrote them.

Fact find

In order to facilitate and maximize results, you must be willing to do some fact finding on the 3 goals and look for potential obstacles you may be up against when aspiring to reach success in these areas. In addition, it's prudent to learn everything possible about your disease, virus, and mental health disorder, or the potential of exposing yourself to the risks.

Being informed about your specific health problems and associated risks is necessary. This entails knowing what the causes are and the statistics surrounding recovery rates. This proactive approach will be beneficial for creating the success strategy for developing the proper protocol to produce maximum results in recovery or prevention.

The only way you can put yourself in the best position for a great outcome is to have valuable information, which includes both positive and negative. List the conditions that are impacting you in a negative way physiologically and mentally and possibly hold you back from reaching those goals. List them in order, from severe to least severe. Be specific.

Goal 1 Anchor1:

____

____

Goal 2 Anchor:

____

____

Goal 3 Anchor:

____

____

Know Your Enemy

Life at times is difficult. When you're facing a crisis, it can take you down a path that can potentially destroy you physically and emotionally. You're at a crossroad, your mind and heart are racing to the point your anxiety shuts you down.

You've lost control of everything, or at least that's your perception, after all perception is reality. Where do you go from here? In order to weaponize your mind and body for the long haul known as life, you must somehow gain control. The same can be said about your body and the little things that can be impacting it in a negative way, like the problems you listed on the previous page. Gain control.

Control, however, is fickle because life is fluid and in a constant state of flux, and change is painful to some degree, even if it's good change. The enemy you are facing is real, even an existential threat, but it can be beaten. Your enemy poses risk factors that can take you out if you don't take heed.

When you're trying to overcome anything that's in control of you, you have to develop a warrior mindset and a strategy to defeat your enemy, because if you don't, you will be left compromised. Minimize your risk factors. Know your enemy. Know your potential risk factors. Plan a way to overcome it.

Add "Why" in front of these problems you listed and create a question for yourself. Write it down below. Answer the questions to the best of your knowledge and dig deep, be specific and honest. If you don't know why, Google the question. Pick one of the answers you find that you feel is probably the answer to your problem.

Problem 1:

Why____

____

Real reason:

____

Problem 2:

Why____

____

REAL reason:

____

Problem 3:

Why____

____

Real reason:

____

Build Your fortress

It takes approximately 4 months to finish an entire fortress, but also recognize that it takes approximately 2-3 million-man hours, 2700 men, working for 100 10-hour days. Perspective and reference are always useful especially when it refers to your body which should be regarded as your own fortress that you'll build, nurture, and maintain for a long prosperous life.

Unfortunately, in today's society, humanity has become their own road block due to their expectations. This is known as the immediate gratification syndrome, which facilitates an environment for mediocrity and failure. This is a problem, but there is always a solution if you look hard and deep. Ask the question, are you worth it? If you answered yes, then make a commitment to yourself to build your own fortress. Unless you have a formula designed for efficient success this can seem like an impossible and daunting task to accomplish.

The fortress you build and maintain will forever protect you because you've weaponized your immune system and your emotional mindset to the degree where diseases, viruses, and mental health disorders can't penetrate it. Make no mistake, this is your foundation that will never let you down. Time to build.

How are you going to do this? Below you will see a guide. Fill in the blanks with your previous obstacle answers. After you have filled it in, Google the sentence you created starting with "how can I….." And write down 3 solutions you found.

Write Reason 1 down below:
How can I work on: ____
Solution 1: ____
Solution 2: ____
Solution 3: ____

Write Reason 2 down below:
How can I work on: ____
Solution 1:____
Solution 2: ____
Solution 3: ____

Write Reason 3 down below:
How can I work on: ____
Solution 1:____
Solution 2: ____
Solution 3: ____

Time to make a PLAN….

Don't overwhelm yourself. So first things first, the number 1 solution is the first and only solution you will focus on in your plan for the first 21 days. After the first 21 days, you will add the second solution into your plan. Once those 21 days end, your last and final solution will be added into your plan for another 21 days.

Part Two

Get Your Mindset Right

The body becomes its function.

Most people don't realize how amazing their body is until they're faced with adversity. It all starts with the mind. Think of your mind as the control tower. When you get your mind right, everything falls into place. Now you're able to access all of the weapons your body has built in itself to help you survive all that life brings. It's a fact that the most powerful thing in the world is thought; however most only tap into a small fraction of its full potential.

So what is the solution? The answer is teaching the body

your need and expectations. You see, the body becomes its
function, which is also known as Wolf's Law.

Through discipline and regimen, the body by its own nature
will adapt to its environment because of the way it was
designed. So, what that means is whatever environment you're
currently in can be changed. This occurrence is known as fight
or flight response. You become what you think. Create the
mindset of a WARRIOR.

Adaptation versus chronic.

There must be a well thought out success strategy for
overcoming adversity. Overcoming and becoming stronger
emotionally and physically requires challenging the mind and
body to get to a better place without being chronically
overwhelmed. You must create an **optional results zone (ORZ)**
where the mind and body can perform to create positive
change. Executing techniques such as intermittent sequencing,
which focuses on specific mental training tactics all the while
remaining in the (ORZ).

This is where the importance of adaptation versus chronic as it
relates to intermittent sequencing becomes an important
factor. Implementing mental training techniques as a regimen
(ex. for 21 days consecutively) then stopping for ten days, once
again returning to the same regimen prove to be most effective
for producing efficient results. The same protocol with regards
to nutritional and exercise regimens apply.

Motivation must be greater than the obstacle.

There is no question that life will test you. You can't get out
without getting your butt kicked. All you can do is plan for it
and do something about it, which is the hard part, because

when everything is going swimmingly human nature lets its guard down unless you are in a mindset of staying on guard and in a preventive mode. Quite honestly, it's difficult for most to be that disciplined; however, it doesn't change the indisputable fact that life will test you. The question is: will you be ready and are you prepared for a pandemic? It's about your motivation to consistently implement a user-friendly strategy for keeping your body's immune system bulletproof to the things that attack your mind and body when your immune system is exposed. The motivation must be greater than life's obstacles.

Moderation is not the key.

The masses are generally wrong, all you must do is reflect on history. No one thought the Wright Brothers would invent the flying machine. When your aspirations are extraordinary, moderation is not the key. It is hard to imagine that being moderate could produce the wrong result, but is true, yet not the absolute truth. You need to do something with extreme behavior to create something extraordinary but know the limit. Knowing when to exercise extreme behavior along with being moderate is a process, and as much a mindset as it is a strategy for controlling physical and emotional stress.

The three components of health: Physical, Mental, and Social

The three components become a stronger health building ally when implemented in conjunction with one another. Leaving one out of the equation compromises overall benefits. In order to create the biggest, most efficient result, a risk analysis must be completed in order to construct a comprehensive regimen where the three components can perform at maximum efficiency specific to each individual need. Take the Health

Triangle Self Assessment and Burn's Depression Checklist provided to get a better idea of where you are and what areas need improvement.

Health Triangle Self Assessment

Healthy: A quality of life utilized by achieving a balanced combination of physical, mental/emotional, and social well-being

Wellness: An overall state of well-being or total health; the ultimate way of life that works to keep the three components of health working together.

Physical Health: Involves keeping your body as fit as possible, practicing good personal hygiene, good nutrition, exercise, proper rest and sleep, and practice good safety habits.

Mental Health: Involves being comfortable with yourself, feeling good about yourself, being able to meet the demands of life, being able to express emotions in healthy ways, and being able to cope with the stress of daily life.

Social Health: Involves how you relate to others, how you choose your friends and activities that you are involved in at home, school, work, and/or leisure.

(Source: www.lessonplanet.com and Dr. David Burnes)

What is Your Level of Wellness?

Directions: Mark the appropriate number on the blank that best categorizes your ranking for each statement below. Add up your numbers and give yourself a subtotal for each section. At the end, add all 3 sub totals for each section to come up with a final total for the entire self-assessment.

Refer to the scoring system at the end to see where you rank.

3=STRONG   2: AVERAGE   1 = WEAK   0= VERY POOR

PHYSICAL HEALTH

_____ I bathe daily. and brush and floss my teeth daily.

_____ I am within 5 pounds of my ideal/desirable weight.

_____ I spend less than 2 hours a day sitting (during free time)

_____My resting heart rate is below 70 beats/minute.

_____ I play/participate in an organized athletic sport/competition.

_____ I do at least 20 minutes of aerobic exercise at least 3 times a week or more

_____ I stretch or do flexibility exercises at least 5-10 minutes every day.

_____ I do strength training exercise for at least 20 minutes for at least 2 times a week or more

_____ I relax at least 15 minutes each day.

_____ I seldom feel tired or run down throughout a normal day.

_____ I get 8 to 10 hours of sleep each night.

_____ I avoid fast food and eat home cooked meals most days.

_____ I eat a balanced diet that includes a variety of foods.

_____ I drink eight cups of water each day.

_____ I eat whole grain bread and cereals and avoid white flour.

_____ I limit my intake of sugar. Have soft drinks less than 3 times a week.

_____ I read the food ingredients lists on packaged food labels to understand the quality of the product.

_____ I avoid the use/abuse non-medicinal drugs, including tobacco and alcohol

_____ I take preventative measures for personal safety.

_____ I analyze health information and products (reading health literature articles, journals, etc.)

___ ___ **SUB TOTAL for PHYSICAL HEALTH (0-60)**

Mental/ Emotional Health

_____I am happy most of the time.
_____I enjoy challenges that help me mentally grow.
_____I can name 3 things I do well.
_____I feel okay about crying and allow myself to do so.
_____I give others sincere compliments.
_____I can accept compliments.
_____I make thoughtful and responsible decisions.
_____I listen to and think about constructive criticism.
_____I ask for help when I need it.
_____I am able to say "no" to people without feeling guilty.
_____I can be satisfied with my effort if I have done my best.
_____I express my thoughts and feelings in a positive manner.
_____I have at least one hobby or interest I pursue and enjoy.
_____I accept responsibility for my actions.
_____I am willing to accept new ideas and try new behaviors I handle setbacks without loss of self-esteem.
_____I am aware of my emotions and manage and express them appropriately.
_____I recognize emotional problems in myself or others and seek help when needed.
_____I feel that my life has meaning and have a sense of control over my life.
_____I successfully manage my stress/frustrations with skill and enjoyment, not letting it become overwhelming.

_____SUBTOTAL for MENTAL / EMOTIONAL HEALTH (0-60)

Social Health

_____I show respect and care for myself and others.
_____I communicate clearly and use good active listening skills with others.
_____I meet people easily and am comfortable entering into conversations with new acquaintances.
_____I continue to participate in an activity even though I don't always get my way.
_____I have at least one or two close friends (develops supportive friendships)
_____I can be assertive and set personal boundaries with family, friends, others, etc.
_____When working in a group, I accept other people's ideas and suggestions.
_____I can say "no" to my friends if they are doing something I do not want to do.
_____I can accept differences in my friends and classmates.
_____I usually have success making friends with females of my age.
_____I usually have success making friends with males of my age.
_____I am comfortable carrying on a conversation with an adult.
_____If I have a problem with someone, I try to work it out (resolves conflicts effectively)
_____I avoid gossiping about people.
_____I seek and lend support when needed.
_____I socialize well with others without the influence of alcohol or other drugs.
_____I understand and accept my own sexuality.
_____I understand the risks of sexually transmitted diseases and pregnancy and take responsibility for my own behavior.
_____I continue growing, learning, and facing new challenges throughout life.
_____I relate to the larger environment (home, community, world) and take a share of the responsibility for it.

_____SUBTOTAL for SOCIAL HEALTH (0-60)

Follow steps on next page to get your score…

TOTALS

______ SUB TOTAL for PHYSICAL HEALTH (0-60)

\+

______ SUB TOTAL for MENTAL HEALTH (0-60)

\+

______ SUB TOTAL for SOCIAL HEALTH (0-60)

\=

______ THE FINAL TOTALS (0-180)

SCORING
165-180 OUTSTANDING
150-164 GREAT
135-149 GOOD
120-134 FAIR
100-119 AVERAGE
75-99 BELOW AVERAGE
50-74 POOR
0-49 NEEDS HELP

Burn's Depression Checklist

		0 = Not At All	1= So me wh at	2= Mo der atel y	3 = A Lot	4= Extre mely
Instructions: Put a check to indicate how much you have experienced each symptom during the past week, including today. Please answer all 25 items.						
Thoughts and Feelings						
1	Feeling sad or down in the dumps					
2	Feeling unhappy or blue					
3	Crying spells or tearfulness					
4	Feeling discouraged					
5	Feeling hopeless					
6	Low self-esteem					
7	Feeling worthless or inadequate					
8	Guilt or shame					
9	Criticizing yourself or blaming others					
10	Difficulty making decisions					
Activities and Personal Relationships						
11	Loss of interest in family, friends or colleagues					
12	Loneliness					
13	Spending less time with family or friends					
14	Loss of motivation					
15	Loss of interest in work or other activities					
16	Avoiding work or other activities					
17	Loss of pleasure or satisfaction in life					
Physical Symptoms						
18	Feeling tired					
19	Difficulty sleeping or sleeping too much					
20	Decreased or increased appetite					
21	Loss of interest in sex					
22	Worrying about your health					
Suicidal Urges						
23	Do you have any suicidal thoughts?					
24	Would you like to end your life?					
25	Do you have a plan for harming yourself?					

Please Total Your Score on Items 1-25 Here:

Total Score	level of Depression
No Depression	0-5
Normal but Unhappy	6-10
Mild Depression	11 - 25
Moderate depression	26-50
Severe depression	51·75
Extreme Depression	76-100

Alkaline versus Acidic

Your physiology is in a state of flux, which simply means it is either in an alkaline or acidic state of being. There are different reasons one's body becomes acidic including: chronic stress, and a diet, especially those that are high in processed foods, gains, sugar to name a few. Lifestyle plays a role. For example if you're a workaholic, stressing your mind and body to an extent it's consistently exhausting. Acid to the body causes inflammation and chronic inflammation can potentially cause major health problems. Changing one's lifestyle and diet can immediately put your body into an alkaline state which staves off disease considering that disease thrives on acid, and without it, it can't harbor itself.

What stresses you out, mentally or physically? _____________

____

Are you eating more healthy foods, or more processed food?

____

Proactive versus inactive

It's easy to succumb to adversity when it's all consuming. It creates a downward spiral taking on a life of its own. When you've arrived at this state it doesn't seem like there's a way out. Motivation has to be greater than the obstacle, but when the motivation has disappeared, there must be some form of discipline to carry you through. Being proactive is the answer, because it's the difference between taking action to control a situation, as opposed to just responding to it after it has happened.

This is a huge distinction. When you're proactive, even if it means producing the wrong result, it is still better than being in a state of apathy. The focus must be on taking baby steps, while also celebrating all the breakthroughs no matter how small.

What's your motivation?__________________________________

____

How will you stay disciplined? __________________________

____

Discipline destroys disappointment

Discipline is the great equalizer, because when you have those moments when you've lost motivation, discipline will carry you through. Real discipline is hard to come by because there's a price you pay. It needs to be earned, and it must be self-induced. It can't be thoroughly instilled by anyone other than you. It takes around thirty days to develop a habit; however, discipline is way more than a habit, it's a lifelong commitment, which is a price most people aren't willing to pay. No one said it would be easy... be prepared.

How will you hold yourself accountable to your discipline?

____

____

____

More is less

Human nature responds to pleasure and pain. When they like something they want more, when they don't like something they want less, even to the point they quit. When you're in a state of emotional and physical repair, realize your immune system is exposed. You must proceed with caution when restoring your health. Keep in mind, in most instances, doing the right thing for the body is counterintuitive. Most people don't trust their instincts, which causes a scenario for worsening and creating a bigger problem. Bottom line, doing more of something generally produces less result, and vice versa. Quality is more useful than quantity in most cases.

What is it you think you are doing that is extreme behavior?

___

Is it a positive or negative in your life?

___

The art of compartmentalization

Life can be all consuming, filled with stress, especially when it becomes chronic. If you don't have the skill set with a strategy to derail the downward spiral, it can send the physiology into what's known as adrenal burnout, which can be fatal. At this point being objective is difficult, yet a rational mind is and must be the priority for the purpose of coming up with a viable solution. Changing the toxic environment you're trapped in requires a smart approach. An immediate way is to break the current cycle of thought and physical state of being. This is a painful, rip off the band-aid approach, but you must wipe the slate clean in order to create a different, more productive life. Most individuals understand the harmful consequences of stress, but stress takes on another level of danger when it becomes toxic to the point where the body completely shuts down. How can you live your life while dealing with all the daily challenges? Compartmentalizing your life on a daily basis is a great option, which simply means divide your lifestyle into sections or categories over a seven day period. Instead of life being all consuming and overwhelming, it's dealt with one day at a time.

Mondays I will focus on/ complete

____

____

Tuesday I will focus on/complete

____

____

Wednesday I will focus on/ complete

____

____

Thursday I will focus on/complete

____

____

Friday I will focus on/ complete

____

____

Saturday I will focus on/complete

____

____

Sunday I will focus on/ complete

____

____

Living in a bubble kills the immune system

No one ever said life wouldn't be dangerous, yet most people live their life in fear. It's a physiological proven fact that when your body perceives a threat it secretes the necessary hormones to protect itself, which is known as fight or flight. Humans are equipped with a clear-thinking mind; however, they must be willing to think for themselves, which is easier said than done, because most individuals suffer from the plight of sheep mentality. In other words, just because it's popular to follow the crowd doesn't mean it's the right thing to do. In fact, it can weaken your immune system as it relates to keeping it strong in the face of overcoming disease, virus, and depression. It's imperative to use common sense and think for yourself, otherwise there could be unintended, dire consequences. Don't kill your immune system.

Are you afraid of life? ___________________

Are you a follower or a leader? ___________________

Do you think for yourself or do you let society think for you? ___________________

Hydration is more than consuming fluid

It's safe to say most individuals understand the importance of hydration, yet most are dehydrated. Most individuals probably equate hydration with the consumption of fluid, which in part is an accurate statement. However not all fluid is of equal value with respect to keeping the body hydrated. Coffee and water are prime examples. Although coffee is mostly water, it is a stimulant and a natural diuretic, thus causing dehydration.

When you drink excess water, it acts as a diuretic, producing the same result as coffee. A simple solution for creating more efficient hydration is to drink fluid containing sodium, such as energy drinks like Gatorade. Simply stated, sodium retains water making it a smart option to use in conjunction with water or coffee. One must also factor in the power of consuming food as it relates to hydration, such as carbohydrates, protein, and fat. For example, consuming a high protein, high fat, low carbohydrate diet produces a natural diuretic effect on the body.

Consequently, when consuming a carbohydrate based diet, your body automatically becomes more hydrated because of the natural profile of that macro inherently having a higher water content. However, this being stated, by eating more carbs doesn't assure proper hydration, because not all carbs are equal, unless you know how to compartmentalize and manipulate macros in a targeted way.

Part 2
Macro Circuit Diet
Manipulating the Macros

What is Macro Circuit Diet?

Macro Circuit Diet is defined by 3 modules: Flush, Restore, and Combo. Each module is a frame of time where macronutrients are prioritized. In addition, modules can change their placement throughout the week determined by individual objectives.

Although each module is independent of one another, they seamlessly integrate throughout each week as a whole creating the Macro effect, otherwise known as Gestalt, where the sum is greater than its parts, this equaling synergy and efficiency.

The beauty of MCD is its simplicity and the ability to produce powerful health results simply by eating the foods you love. To understand how MCD works is to fully understand how powerful food can be when eaten in proper combinations, as well in complete harmony with the normal function of physiology. A proper diet doesn't need gimmicks or tricks for it to work. MCD is designed with that understanding.

The Power of Macros

Just exactly what are protein, carbs, and fat? Most people have a general idea, but not specifically. For most, there's confusion mainly because of all the diets out there touting their uniqueness, but not really highlighting any basic mechanics of how it all works. When this happens, the consumer becomes mindless, which works for a large segment of the population who have a sheep mentality. You certainly don't have to be a nutrition guru, but you should have a proper, yet simple understanding of the food that is responsible for providing 100% of the energy to your body.

Protein, Carbs, Fats: The roles they play

Protein is responsible for making enzymes, hormones, and other body chemicals. It is an important building block of bones, muscles, cartilage, skin and blood. Generally, the body needs relatively large amounts of protein. **Carbohydrates** provide the body with energy broken down from simple sugars including glucose, fructose, sucrose, and lactose, in addition to many complex carbohydrates like starch, which are made up of sugar molecules joined together.

Fats are made chiefly of triglycerides, each molecule of which contain three fatty acids. Dietary fat supplies humans with essential fatty acids, such as linoleic and linolenic. Fat also regulates cholesterol metabolism, and is a precursor of prostaglandins.

Protein Is Not Stored

By definition, protein is any class of nitrogenous organic compounds that consist of large molecules composed of one or more long chains of amino acids and are an essential part of all living organisms. It's a structural building block in your body for everything, including muscle, hair, collagen etc. Interestingly, as complex as protein is, it doesn't have the specialized cellular capacity to be efficiently stored within the body. Here in lies the very reason why you need to regularly intake protein, otherwise your body will cannibalize on itself breaking down its own muscle tissue to get nutrients.

Carbs Are Not Always the Best Energy Source

By definition, carbs are any of a large group of compounds occurring in foods and living tissues including sugars, starch and cellulose. They contain hydrogen and oxygen in the same ratio as water (2:1) and typically can be broken down to release energy in the body. Although a formidable source, carbs aren't always the best option for energy because of how it releases within your body. The term good and bad carbs are used in the nutrition industry, mainly as a sexy buzz word, in addition to creating distinction. The good carb simply means it's a complex carbohydrate, which is a long chain sugar that takes longer to release in the body. Bad carb are considered a simple carbohydrate which is a shorter chain of sugar that releases in the body much quicker. If too many simple carbohydrates are ingested at one time, the body is not capable of utilizing all of the energy released, causing the body to store the overage as a fat known as triglycerides, which can negatively impact HDL and LDL cholesterol.

Fat Is Not the Culprit

When your body has an overage of calories that it can't use right away, they're converted into triglycerides, that are stored in your fat cells. Later, hormones release triglycerides for energy between meals. In addition, fat serves as a backup source of energy to fuel your workout when carbohydrates aren't available. Fat is an essential part of your diet. It provides energy, absorbs certain nutrients and maintains your core body temperature; however, fat plays an even bigger role. It can be very powerful nutritional tool when used properly. For instance, it can be used to control sugar. In addition, eating a diet that has a higher fat content can also make your body more efficient in storing less body fat. High blood sugar levels, caused from ingesting too many carbohydrates (sugar) can create havoc and be unhealthy. Your body can only store so many carbs before it converts it to a triglyceride. Unlike dietary fat, excess triglycerides in your bloodstream are dangerous fats. Consequently, eating fat as a part of your everyday diet can be very healthy because of its powerful positive interaction with sugar, which achieves a few things. It stabilizes, even eliminating fluctuations of energy, which also reduces hunger.

Calories Are Key

What is a calorie? Most people don't really know, which makes the calorie somewhat of an enigma in terms of how it impacts physiology. For years, there has been a debate over whether or not all calories are equal. The debate will invariably continue on, mainly by those who don't really know unless they've been in the trenches with firsthand experience. If you really want to know how calories impact the body, ask a world level bodybuilder. Their bodies are their laboratory where experimenting with calories and determining how well they perform is normal protocol. All calories are a unit of heat that indicate the amount of energy that foods will produce in the body. Eating a calorie is nothing more than a transference of heat that fuels the body to make it move and think.

Compartmentalization Is Your Secret Weapon

Knowing how to use calories in your diet can be the difference between reaching your full athletic potential if you are an athlete or reversing heart disease if your health is failing. This is a broad application with an even bigger impact. The diet components which include protein, carbs, and fat that specifically need to be manipulated are called macronutrients. Like everything, there's a process and method to the madness. In order to get the most out of your diet, you must first understand how to most effectively utilize protein, carbs, and fat in order to supercharge your body's metabolism. To put it more succinctly, if certain foods are combined with one another on certain days of the week, they become a powerhouse making your body much more effective in the way it performs.

Change the Way You See Your Food

Most people are not in control when it comes to food, and because of the emotional connection, many are enslaved, even held hostage. People eat food for different reasons, including to comfort themselves when sad. There are those who stress eaters and others who are just overwhelmingly addicted. Simply put, most people live to eat instead of eating to live.

Eat the Foods You Love

Lose weight, get healthy, and reverse heart disease one bite at a time. It's hard to believe you can eat anything you want, lose weight, reverse heart disease and become healthier. It's true and I'm a walking testimonial, with doctor's verification. It's a safe bet and assumption there will be a whole host of so-called experts and critics scoffing at this diet, but that's normal. Bodybuilders know what it takes to get the most out of nutrition because their bodies are an ongoing experiment. They understand nutrition in a way that even most who claim they are experts can't. Here is the truth. If you really understand how to manipulate nutrition, you have at your disposal one of the most powerful weapons.

Breaking Points

"Too hot, too cold, I'm tired, I have a headache, there's a storm coming." There's an old saying that goes: Excuses are like buttholes. Everybody has one and they all stink. Individuals, for various reasons have a tendency of sabotaging their own results. Anything you do long-term requires a tremendous amount of discipline, even more importantly passion, motivation, and belief. Breaking points are a normal part of anything long-term, and are necessary, which will only build strength and character, but you have to be willing to endure the process.

What's Your Number?

In order to create a formula for the purpose of producing targeted results, there must be an equation. That's how things are measured in order to determine its effectiveness. With regard to caloric intake and how it impacts your state of condition, understanding that we all have a number is imperative. Your caloric number at times will be static as well as fluctuating, depending on whether weight loss, weight maintenance, or weight gain is the objective. Most experts in the nutrition industry will claim that you should stop eating after 6pm because it leads to added weight gain. It's not bad information; however, it is inaccurate. Remember, it's all about how many calories you need that coincides with your specific objectives. Bodybuilders know this at times waking up in the middle of the night to eat. Enough said!

Why Triglycerides Are Your Ace in the Hole

Triglycerides generally have a negative connotation, but there's more to a triglyceride than meets the eye. By definition, triglycerides are a type of fat found in your blood, which your body uses for energy. A triglyceride enters your body in various forms, including foods that have a natural fat content. However, dietary fat consumption does not affect triglyceride levels unlike glucose, in other words, carbohydrates. Nevertheless, your body stores excess calories, mostly sugar, as a triglyceride. It's imperative that you have triglycerides for good health. However, if they get too elevated it can cause major health problems.

The positive side of a triglyceride, and one of its main purposes is that when you need energy, such as in between meals, hormones will automatically release them into your body. They're like a backup built-in generator that is always ready at a moment's notice. But like any other powerful weapon, there is an up and downside to a triglyceride depending upon how it is used.

Eating More Times a Day Is Not the Final Answer

It has not been scientifically validated that eating smaller meals more frequently throughout the day is more beneficial than eating larger meals less frequently. In fact, it can slow down the fat burning process. At the end of the day, if you eat the right number of calories, your body will respond. The body has an amazing capability of adapting and providing necessary calories as needed. However, understanding how to manipulate the components of nutrition can dramatically improve metabolic activity. For example, eating foods that require more energy to break down, causes thermogenesis, which is defined as the production of heat. In other words, the amount of energy you burn depends on the food you eat. This is known as the thermic effect of food which improves the way your body feels and performs. It should be noted that of all the foods you eat, protein is the most metabolically expensive—it takes more energy to break down, digest, and put to use as opposed to carbohydrates or fat. Up to 30 percent of the calories you eat from protein are burned during the digestion and processing of those foods.

That is one of the main reasons why diets with protein are so great; the more protein you eat, the more calories you burn. Carbohydrates and fats on the other hand are less metabolically active, with carbohydrates burning about 6 to 8 percent of its calories during digestion and processing, and fats about 4 percent burned, despite being the highest in calories and great for your testosterone levels. The lesson to learn from this is that less rather than more can garner bigger benefits. To top all this off, eating fewer times per day triggers your body to secrete bigger amounts of digestive enzymes and bile, which breaks down fat into usable energy making your metabolism more efficient.

Neither Man nor Woman Can Live on Carbs Alone

There is no argument that carbohydrates are an adequate source of energy, but the truth is, if you only ate them, you'd eventually die off of what's known as protein starvation. However, if you only ate protein the opposite is true. Let us identify why. First and most importantly, the structure and function of our bodies depend on proteins, and the regulation of the body's cells, tissues, and organs cannot exist without them. Secondly, muscles, skin, bones and other parts of the human body contain significant amounts of protein, including enzymes, hormones and antibodies. Protein also works as a neurotransmitter. Hemoglobin, a carrier of oxygen in the blood, is protein. Wait, there is more. Protein is highly adaptive and transformative.

Unlike carbohydrates, protein can adapt when necessary, as an example through the process of converting carbons within its own structure into glucose, which is the only energy in which the brain can function. Paul Harvey used to say at the end of his radio show, "Now you know the rest of the story."

My Story

My name is Leo Costa Jr. I am a former world-level bodybuilder who had three strokes in three weeks that paralyzed my right side. It has now been six years since the event, where I have now regained 100% of my motor skill functions. Doctors call me a miracle. One major factor in my recovery has been my implementation and execution of nutrition. Because of stroke risk factors, it was crucial I made immediate lifestyle changes, one being to lose a significant amount of weight, and because of blockages in my arteries, it was suggested by my doctor to go on medication.

This is when I made the decision **not** to follow my doctor's recommendation, and instead make some changes with my diet. Here's the great news. After implementing my new eating strategy for one year, I returned to the doctor for a yearly checkup. In his surprise and amazement, he said I had significantly reduced the blockage in my arteries. His next question was telling, which became my inspiration for developing MCD. He asked, "What did you do?"

MCD is defined by modules, meaning there are specific days of the week where certain combinations of foods are consumed for the directed purpose of creating a powerful physiological impact, using macronutrients as the vehicle for delivery.

The Misconception

Ask five different so-called experts on the best diet to follow and more than likely you will get five different opinions. There is no doubt there is more than one effective diet on the market that can produce results, as well as appear to be unique and different, but they are more uniquely similar than different. Occasionally, you will find a diet that really does work, but most are short-lived mainly because of restricted complexity. Here is the truth. If you want a diet that produces long-term results, implement something that is simple to use.

Step One of Macro Circuit Diet: Understand the Diet Process

Flush (Monday): You will begin a liquid fast for 24hrs, which will then transition you into Restore.

Restore (Tuesday through Friday): A specific designed style of eating is implemented for 4 days starting Tuesday and ending Friday, before transitioning you into Combo.

Combo (Saturday through Sunday): Any combination of food is allowed, before transitioning you back into another week starting with Flush.

Step Two of Macro Circuit Diet: Finding the Right Calories for Weight Management Objectives

MCD has three specific calorie categories: Weight Loss, Weight Maintenance and Weight Gain. There are calorie ranges for males and females depending on their weight management objectives. These three categories will apply to both males and females, but with some differences. Men, because of their ability to produce testosterone, naturally carry more muscle mass requiring more calories to maintain the body.

Below is a calorie breakdown in the three categories for men and women:

Men Weight Loss (calorie decrease) 1,500 calories
Men Weight Maintenance 1,800 calories
Men Weight Gain (calorie increase) 2,500 calories
Women Weight Loss (calorie decrease) 1,000 calories
Women Weight Maintenance 1,300 calories
Women Weight Gain (calorie increase) 1,800 calories

MCD Implementation (Modules)

Flush - This module is a 24-hour fast. It technically begins at the end of Combo module where only liquids are consumed. Implementing the Flush module is powerful. The intention of a proper liquid fast is to facilitate the process of cleansing the body, which produces significant results, including short-term weight loss, detoxification, and improved organ and gland function. To maximize this module, it is suggested to only consume water, any fruit juice, black coffee, teas, and broth. It is a good way to reboot and re energize the mind and body, which will enhance performance of the other two modules.

When starting Flush, it is imperative that you begin as early in the morning, as possible and consume liquids throughout the whole day. Do not be concerned about the calories in the juices because in 24 hours it will go right through your body. If you do not begin to push liquids in your system as soon as possible, you will hold water and eliminate the flush benefits.

Restore - This module lasts 4 consecutive days or 96 hours beginning at the conclusion of the Flush module. Restore is a specifically designed style of eating and is considered one of the best ways to eat for overall health. It is considered a very safe and effective way to eat for lowering inflammation in the body, losing body fat, reducing cravings, eliminating edema, and reversing heart disease. In essence, the diet consists of meats, fish, vegetables, nuts, leafy greens, and seeds, which is the Paleo diet, or also known as the Caveman diet.

Combo - This module lasts 48 hours, or any two consecutive days. It begins after the Restore module has concluded. In this module all macros (protein, carbs, fat) are available for consumption in any combination desired, including processed foods, junk food, etc. If you notice you are feeling sluggish, or exhausted it is because you are consuming too much sugar and in order to make your energy levels more consistent you need to increase your fat intake. Examples of high fat foods are; cheeseburger, avocado, dark chocolate, nuts, cheese.

Kitchen Tricks

Kitchen Trick # 1: People eat with their eyes and habits they develop. First, put low calorie foods towards the front of the fridge, so they can be grabbed first. Have a variety of these foods available, including all three macros, and ensure they are colorful.

Kitchen Trick # 2: To keep from overeating, store foods in glass containers that are based on a serving size, which can be easily determined by simply making a fist and putting your fist over food. If a food portion can be seen sticking out anywhere around the fist, that is exceeding an average serving size. Using a fist for selecting portion sizes when plating food or eating out is a valuable guideline.

MCD Simple Tricks

When in doubt, perhaps when traveling, or out of your normal eating environment or routine, yet you still want to follow your MCD to its letter, remember three essential food groups: meat, vegetables, fruit. Although there are additional foods in the Restore Module, eating the three essential food groups will always ensure you are staying on the right path.

Fist It

If you want exact results, you have to be exact. This can be largely challenging. It is recommended on MCD to always weigh your food with a scale as this is the only way you can achieve exact results, while also keeping you highly accountable.

Although this strategy is ideal, it can be inconvenient and user unfriendly, but not to worry, as there is a simple solution, which is your fist. Your fist can be very valuable and surprisingly accurate in determining the caloric value of food. Here's how it works: make a fist.

When you don't have a scale, your fist replaces the scale, **always** equating to an average serving size, which equals 4 ounces. To emphasize, always using your fist as the average serving size, eventually gets you exact results.

Here is an example of a real-life scenario. You're at a restaurant and you order your food. Position your fist a half inch over each food portion. As long as the food portion does not stick out anywhere around the fist, that is considered an average serving size, which is 4 ounces.

The next step is simple math. You will have to research how many calories are in an ounce of the food you are eating. Multiply the calories in an ounce of the food you are eating to the average serving size (your fist), which is 4 ounces (calorie per ounce times 4). You will then get an estimate of how many calories you are eating. Do this with each food choice on your plate, and you will get the estimated count of how many total calories are on your plate.

MCD Caloric Values

Unless you're a top caliber bodybuilder or a nutritionist, it's pretty much a full- time job knowing the exact calories of each food group. One of the objectives of MCD is simplifying something as complex as knowing with accuracy the calorie count of food groups, without sacrificing accuracy.

Index Number

Here's the simple MCD solution. The first step is to pick a food group. For the purpose of the exercise, we will use red meat. Find the red meat that has the highest calories per ounce. Now find the red meat with the lowest calories per ounce. Add those two numbers together and divide by two. The answer is considered the index number for the red meat food group.

In other words, the index number which applies to each food group will always be used as the default number to calculate calories. As with using the fist as an average serving size, the index number used each and every time will produce accurate information.

Cardio Walking

MCD is one of three training components that stands on its own merit producing immediate and ongoing sustainable results. However, when incorporating other training components simultaneously such as cardio walking, which also stands on its own merit, creates a positive compounding effect.

Cardio Calorie Counting Made Simple

Ideally, it's important to know your heart rate when performing cardio walking; however, it is not necessary with MCD because of a simple formula factoring a static number determining average calories burned per minute, which is six calories. To put this into perspective, doing 30 minutes of cardio walking will burn 180 calories.

MCD Your Way

Instead of requiring individuals to compromise their lifestyle to make their diet work for them, MCD has been constructed to adjust around individual lifestyles. The modules in this diet have a broad scope of application, and can be easily adjusted for the purpose of reversing heart disease and inflammation in the body. In addition facilitating pinpoint accuracy for weight loss, athletic performance, improving performance of vitamin supplementation, and improving prescribed medication.

Why Flip Your Metabolism

Humans are the same but different, and so are their metabolisms. Utilizing both metabolisms at some point throughout a diet regimen is highly beneficial, even necessary. Simply put, some individuals, because of their genetic makeup, perform more efficiently utilizing glucose (sugar) metabolism as its main energy source, while others perform more efficiently utilizing the free fatty acid (fat) metabolism. Generally, the reason for this occurrence is due to glucose intolerance, where the individual's physiology is sensitive to sugar in a negative way causing irritation, which can potentially cause a whole host of health problems.

Conversely, there are those individuals who are pre-diabetic, or suffer from type 2 diabetes. In most cases, utilizing the free fatty acid diet is necessary due to the fact that the individual's physiology is unable to produce enough insulin which is responsible for using glucose (sugar) to supply the body with energy, or to store it for future use. In this example, free fatty acid metabolism is a viable option and many times an alternative to having doctor prescribed medication.

Parting Note

I know that if you follow MCD and really give it 100%, it is going to be one of the best decisions of your life, as it was and still is for me. For now, as my great friend and mentor Pat Biele always said, "Onward and Upward."

-Leo Costa Jr

Caloric Intake

<u>Men</u>

Weight Loss: 1,500 calories

Weight Maintenance: 1,800 calories

Weight Gain: 2,500 calories

<u>Women</u>

Weight Loss: 1,000 calories

Weight Maintenance: 1,300 calories

Weight Gain: 1,800 calories

Note: Above are caloric intake suggestions that are based on individual goals. Sometimes the number may have to vary to achieve your desired result. If so, you may need to either add or subtract 300-500 calories to the original caloric intake suggestion.

<u>Macro Circuit Quick Start</u>

1,000 Calorie Meal Plan

These meal plans are for those people who don't have the time to cook meals and need that quick start.

MONDAY BREAKFAST: (EXAMPLE 1)	MONDAY BREAKFAST: (EXAMPLE 2)
HOT BROTH	ORANGE JUICE
• 12 OZ BEEF BROTH, HEATED	• 12 OZ ORANGE JUICE (NO PULP)
LUNCH:	LUNCH:
APPLE JUICE	GRAPE JUICE
• 12 OZ APPLE JUICE	• 12 OZ GRAPE JUICE
DINNER:	DINNER:
CRANBERRY JUICE	TOMATO JUICE
• 12 OZ CRANBERRY JUICE	• 12 OZ TOMATO JUICE
SNACK:	SNACK:
WATER	VEGETABLE JUICE
• 12 OZ WATER	• 12 OZ VEGETABLE JUICE

<u>Reminder:</u> These are 2 examples of what your Mondays will look like. DO NOT FOLLOW THIS PLAN.

Things You Can Have During Your Flush: (Calories for 8 fl ounces)

- Coconut Water (46 Calories)

- Water (0 Calories)

- Carrot Juice (94 Calories)

- Apple Juice (105 Calories)

- Orange Juice (115 Calories)

- Grape Juice (152 Calories)

- Vegetable Juice (50 Calories)

- Pomegranate Juice (140 Calories)

- Tomato Juice (41 Calories)

- Grapefruit Juice (102 Calories)

- Cranberry Juice (116 Calories)

- Chicken Broth (41 Calories)

- Beef Broth (10 Calories)

- Tea (nothing added) (2.4 Calories)

- Coffee (nothing added) (1.8 Calories)

Note: This is a 24-hour fast. No food is to be consumed during this time. It is advised to only choose from the options above. Stay within your caloric intake. This meal plan is just an EXAMPLE of what your Mondays should look like.

TUESDAY BREAKFAST:

WEDNESDAY BREAKFAST:

TROPICAL SKIN CLEANSING SMOOTHIE
- ¾ CUP SPINACH
- ½ CUP COCONUT WATER
- ½ CUP PINEAPPLE
- 2 TBSP AVOCADO

CHIA SEED PAPAYA SHAKE
- 1 ¼ CUP ALMOND MILK
- 2 TBSP CHIA SEEDS
- ½ CUP CUBED PAPAYA

TUESDAY LUNCH:

SALMON
- 6 OZ PINK SALMON

STRAWBERRIES
- 1 CUP STRAWBERRIES

WEDNESDAY LUNCH:

ZUCCHINI
- 1 2/3 LARGE ZUCCHINI

BEEF TENDERLOIN
- 4 OZ BEEF TENDERLOIN

TUESDAY DINNER:

COD
- 8 OZ COD

CARROTS
- 1 CUP BABY CARROTS

WEDNESDAY DINNER:

CORN
- 1 LARGE EAR CORN

SALMON
- 3 OZ PINK SALMON

TUESDAY SNACK:

BANANA & ALMOND BUTTER
- 1 MEDIUM BANANA
- 2 TBSP ALMOND BUTTER

BROCCOLI
- 6 OZ BROCCOLI

WEDNESDAY SNACK:

TURKEY LETTUCE ROLLUPS
- 6 OUTER LETTUCE LEAVES
- 6 SLICES DELI TURKEY

BANANA
- 1 MEDIUM BANANA

Thursday and Friday on next page…

QUICK START: RESTORE	*THURSDAY-FRIDAY: 1,000 CALORIES*
THURSDAY BREAKFAST	**FRIDAY BREAKFAST**
HIGH PROTEIN OMELET • 3 LARGE EGG WHITES • 2 LARGE EGGS • 3 TBSP BARBECUE SAUCE	BANANA EGG PANCAKES • 1 MEDIUM BANANA • 2 LARGE EGGS BLEND AND COOK.
THURSDAY LUNCH:	FRIDAY LUNCH:
SALMON • 3 OZ PINK SALMON	CHICKEN SALAD • 4 OZ CHICKEN BREAST • 2 TBSP LIGHT MAYONNAISE
	FRIDAY DINNER:
TOMATO SOUP • ½ CAN OF TOMATO SOUP • ½ CAN OF WATER	SALMON • 4 OZ SALMON
THURSDAY DINNER:	FRIDAY SNACK:
CHICKEN & AVOCADO SALAD • 1 CAN OF CANNED CHICKEN • ½ AVOCADO • 4 LARGE LEAFS OF LETTUCE	BANANA & ALMOND BUTTER • 1 BANANA • 2 OZ ALMOND BUTTER
THURSDAY SNACK:	
APPLE & ALMOND BUTTER • 1 MEDIUM APPLES • 2 TBSP ALMOND BUTTER	

QUICK START: RESTORE	*SUBSTITUTE MEAL PLANS: 1,000 CALORIES*
(SUBSTITUTE 1) BREAKFAST:	**(SUBSTITUTE 2) BREAKFAST:**

STRAWBERRY WATERMELON SMOOTHIE	DENVER OMELET
• ½ TBSP LIME JUICE	• 2 EXTRA LARGE EGG
• 1 CUP WATERMELON BALLS	• 2 SLICES HAM
• ½ CUP UNTHAWED STRAWBERRIES	
• ¾ TSP MAPLE SYRUP	

LUNCH:	**LUNCH:**

DEVILED EGG SALAD	STEAK
• 2 EXTRA LARGE EGGS	• 2 OZ BEEF TENDERLOIN
• 1 TBSP MAYONNAISE	• ¼ TBSP OLIVE OIL

	DINNER:

SAUTEED KALE	BALSAMIC CHICKEN
• ¼ CUP CHOPPED KALE	• 1 TSP ITALIAN SALAD DRESSING
• ½ TBSP OLIVE OIL	• 1 TBSP BALSAMIC VINEGAR
	• ½ TBSP GRAMS HONEY
	• 5 OZ CHICKEN BREAST
	• ½ TBSP OLIVE OIL

DINNER:	

GRILLED STEAK	MIXED VEGGIES
• 5 OZ SIRLOIN STEAK	• 4 OZ ASPARAGUS
• ¾ TSP OLIVE OIL	• ¼ CUP CHERRY TOMATOES
• ½ TBSP BALSAMIC VINEGAR	• 1.5 OZ CARROTS
	• 1 MEDIUM ZUCCHINI

	SNACK:

ZUCCHINI	GRAPES
• 1 MEDIUM ZUCCHINI	• 2 CUPS GRAPES

SNACK:	

TURKEY LETTUCE ROLL UPS	
• 2 OUTER LETTUCE LEAVES	
• 2 SLICES DELI TURKEY	

ALMOND BUTTER & CELERY	
• 2 TBSP ALMOND BUTTER	
• 2 STALKS LARGE CELERY	

<u>Note:</u> Above are two full day "substitute" meal plans that can be used to interchange any day in Restore week (Tuesday through Friday). Choose one substitute meal plan and substitute it in for any day you choose.

FOOD ITEM	AVERAGE SERVING SIZE	CALORIES
PROTEIN		
HAMBURGER PATTY	3.5 OZ	235 CAL
TRI TIP	3.5 OZ	182 CAL
PORK CUTLET	3.5 OZ	231 CAL
CHICKEN	4 OZ	190 CAL
BEEF NEW YORK STRIP STEAK	4 OZ	220 CAL
BABY BACK RIBS	3 OZ	270 CAL
PORK SIRLOIN	3 OZ	168 CAL
BEEF RIBEYE STEAK	6 OZ	450 CAL
SALMON	3 OZ	200 CAL
HALIBUT	3 OZ	107 CAL
FRIED EGG	1 LARGE EGG	92 CAL
BOILED EGG	1 LARGE EGG	77 CAL
SCRAMBLED EGG	1 LARGE EGG	101 CAL
CARBOHYDRATES		
BANANA	1 MEDIUM BANANA	104 CAL
APPLE	1 MEDIUM APPLE	80 CAL
ORANGE	1 FRUIT	69 CAL
SPAGHETTI WITH MEAT SAUCE	10 OZ	286 CAL
CHICKEN ALFREDO PASTA	8.14 OZ	321 CAL
WHITE RICE	1 CUP	205 CAL
BROWN RICE	1 CUP	216 CAL
BLACK BEANS	½ CUP	90 CAL
REFRIED BEANS	½ CUP	125 CAL
PINTO BEANS	½ CUP	144 CAL
BROCCOLI	1 CUP	65 CAL
GREEN BEANS	1 CUP	25 CAL
CORN	4 OZ	153 CAL
WHOLE WHEAT BREAD	1 SLICE	69 CAL
WHITE BREAD	1 SLICE	120 CAL
SOURDOUGH BREAD	1 SLICE	120 CAL
RESTAURANTS		
IN N OUT BURGER WITH ONION	1 SERVING	390 CAL

MCDONALDS CHEESEBURGER	1 SERVING	300 CAL
TACO BELL CRUNCHY SUPREME TACO	1 SERVING	190 CAL
TACO BELL BEAN BURRITO	1 SERVING	370 CAL
EL POLLO LOCO AL CARBON CHICKEN TACOS	1 SERVING	160 CAL
JAMBA JUICE ACAI PRIMO FRUIT BOWL	1 SERVING	540 CAL
CARL'S JR SPICY CHICKEN SANDWICH	1 SERVING	460 CAL
SUBWAY HAM SANDWICH 6 INCH	1 SERVING	450 CAL
PANERA BREAD STRAWBERRY POPPYSEED CHICKEN SALAD	1 SERVING	350 CAL
RED LOBSTER STARTER SAMPLER	1 SERVING	620 CAL
OLIVE GARDEN CHICKEN ALFREDO FETTUCCINE	1 SERVING	500 CAL
RED ROBIN WINGS	1 SERVING	1,023 CAL
APPLEBEE'S TRIPLE BACON BURGER	1 SERVING	1,190 CAL

<u>Note:</u> Above is an example of the same but not all food items allowed in Combo. Remember you can eat anything you want in Combo (Saturday and Sunday) as long as you stay within your targeted caloric intake.

QUICK START: COMBO	*SATURDAY- SUNDAY: 1,000 CALORIES*
SATURDAY BREAKFAST: • ½ CUP OATMEAL (PLAIN) (150 CALORIES) • 70 CAL WHEAT BREAD (70 CALORIES) • 1 TSP BUTTER (34 CALORIES)	**SUNDAY BREAKFAST:** • 1 BUTTERMILK PANCAKE (175 CALORIES) • 2 TBSP LITE SYRUP (53 CALORIES)
SATURDAY LUNCH: • GRILLED CHEESE SANDWICH (257 CALORIES) • 7 COOL RANCH CHIPS (88 CALORIES)	**SUNDAY LUNCH:** • IN N OUT BURGER (195 CALORIES) • 1.5 OZ FRIES (126 CALORIES)
SATURDAY DINNER: • 7 OZ STOUFFER LASAGNA (277 CALORIES) • 1 OZ CORN BREAD SLICE (67 CALORIES)	**SUNDAY DINNER:** • 1 CHEESE PIZZA SLICE (272 CALORIES)
SATURDAY SNACK: • 1 SUGAR FREE JELLO CUP (5 CALORIES) • .5 OZ POPCORN (50 CALORIES)	**SUNDAY SNACK:** • 1 MEDIUM GLAZED DONUT (192 CALORIES)
TOTAL: 998 CALORIES	TOTAL: 1,012 CALORIES

<u>Note:</u> In Combo you can eat ANY food, but stay in your caloric intake!

Macro Circuit Quick Start

1,300 Calorie Meal Plan

These meal plans are for those people who don't have the time to cook meals and need that quick start.

MONDAY BREAKFAST: (EXAMPLE 1)	MONDAY BREAKFAST: (EXAMPLE 2)
HOT BROTH	ORANGE JUICE
• 12 OZ BEEF BROTH, HEATED	• 12 OZ ORANGE JUICE (NO PULP)
LUNCH:	LUNCH:
APPLE JUICE	GRAPE JUICE
• 12 OZ APPLE JUICE	• 12 OZ GRAPE JUICE
DINNER:	DINNER:
CRANBERRY JUICE	TOMATO JUICE
• 12 OZ CRANBERRY JUICE	• 12 OZ TOMATO JUICE
SNACK:	SNACK:
WATER	VEGETABLE JUICE
• 12 OZ WATER	• 12 OZ VEGETABLE JUICE

<u>Reminder:</u> These are 2 examples of what your Mondays will look like. DO NOT FOLLOW THIS PLAN.

Things You Can Have During Your Flush: (Calories for 8 fl ounces)

- Coconut Water (46 Calories)

- Water (0 Calories)

- Carrot Juice (94 Calories)

- Apple Juice (105 Calories)

- Orange Juice (115 Calories)

- Grape Juice (152 Calories)

- Vegetable Juice (50 Calories)

- Pomegranate Juice (140 Calories)

- Tomato Juice (41 Calories)

- Grapefruit Juice (102 Calories)

- Cranberry Juice (116 Calories)

- Chicken Broth (41 Calories)

- Beef Broth (10 Calories)

- Tea (nothing added) (2.4 Calories)

- Coffee (nothing added) (1.8 Calories)

Note: This is a 24-hour fast. No food is to be consumed during this time. It is advised to only choose from the options above. Stay within your caloric intake. This meal plan is just an EXAMPLE of what your Mondays should look like.

TUESDAY BREAKFAST:

KALE AND EGG CUP
- 3 EXTRA LARGE EGGS
- 8 OZ KALE
- 1 TBSP OLIVE OIL

BLUEBERRIES
- 1 CUP BLUEBERRIES

TUESDAY LUNCH:

SEARED STRIP STEAK
- 6 OZ BEEF STEAK
- 1 TSP OLIVE OIL

TUESDAY DINNER:

GRILLED CHICKEN
- 6 OZ CHICKEN BREAST

BRUSSEL SPROUTS
- 1 CUP BRUSSELS SPROUTS

TUESDAY SNACK:

SALAD
- 2 CUPS SALAD
- 2 TBSP RANCH

CARROTS
- 1 CUP BABY CARROTS

WEDNESDAY BREAKFAST:

SAUSAGE AND EGG WHITE SCRAMBLE
- 3 EGG WHITES
- 2 OZ SAUSAGE
- 1 TBSP OLIVE OIL

ORANGE
- 1 ORANGE

WEDNESDAY LUNCH:

CHICKEN, SPINACH, AND STRAWBERRY SALAD
- 4 OZ CHICKEN BREAST
- 6 CUPS SPINACH
- 1 CUP HALVED STRAWBERRIES
- 4 TBSP BALSAMIC VINEGAR

WEDNESDAY DINNER:

BEEF TOP SIRLOIN
- 4 OZ BEEF SIRLOIN

ZUCCHINI
- 2 ½ LARGE ZUCCHINI

WEDNESDAY SNACK:

ALMONDS
- 1 OZ ALMONDS (23 KERNELS)

Thursday and Friday on next page…

QUICK START: RESTORE

THURSDAY BREAKFAST:

EGGS

- 3 LARGE EGGS

BACON

- 3 STRIPS BACON

THURSDAY LUNCH:

BARBECUE CHICKEN

- 6 OZ CHICKEN BREAST
- 2 TBSP BARBECUE SAUCE

BROCCOLI

- 8 OZ BROCCOLI

THURSDAY DINNER:

CHICKEN, SPINACH, AND STRAWBERRY SALAD

- 2 OZ CHICKEN BREAST
- 3 CUPS SPINACH
- ½ CUP STRAWBERRIES
- 2 TBSP BALSAMIC VINEGAR

THURSDAY SNACK:

TURKEY LETTUCE ROLL UP

- 2 OUTER LETTUCE LEAVES
- 2 SLICES DELI TURKEY
- 2 CUP BABY CARROTS

THURSDAY- FRIDAY: 1,300 CALORIES

FRIDAY BREAKFAST:

SAUSAGE AND EGG SCRAMBLE

- 3 EXTRA LARGE EGGS
- 2 OZ SAUSAGE

FRIDAY LUNCH:

MEATBALLS

- 4 OZ GROUND BEEF MEATBALLS
- 1 CUP TOMATO SOUP

FRIDAY DINNER:

SCALLOPS

- 9 OZ SCALLOPS
- 2 CUPS GREEN BEANS

BANANA

- 2 BANANAS

FRIDAY SNACK:

SPINACH SALAD

- 5 CUPS SPINACH
- 2 LARGE SCALLIONS
- 2 TBSP RANCH DRESSING

QUICK START: RESTORE	*SUBSTITUTE MEAL PLANS: 1,300 CALORIES*
(SUBSTITUTE 1) BREAKFAST:	(SUBSTITUTE 2) BREAKFAST:
EGGS	GARLIC OMELET
• 6 LARGE EGGS • 2 BACON STRIPS	• 4 LARGE EGGS • ½ TSP GARLIC POWDER • ½ TBSP OLIVE OIL
APPLE	ORANGE
• 1 APPLE	• 1 FRUIT ORANGE
LUNCH:	LUNCH:
BEEF TENDERLOIN	STEAK AND CORN
• 4 OZ BEEF TENDERLOIN	• 6 OZ FLANK STEAK • 1 CUP CORN
DINNER:	DINNER:
SHRIMP	CHICKEN
• 6 OZ SHRIMP	• 4 OZ GRILLED CHICKEN
BROCCOLI	TOMATO SOUP
• 2 CUPS BROCCOLI	• 1 CAN TOMATO SOUP • 1 CUP WATER • MIX, BOIL AND ENJOY!
SNACK:	SNACK:
GRAPE	TURKEY LETTUCE ROLLUPS
• 2 CUPS GRAPES	• 2 OUTER LETTUCE LEAVES • 2 SLICES DELI TURKEY
	CARROTS
	• 1 CUP BABY CARROTS

<u>Note:</u> Above are two full day "substitute" meal plans that can be used to interchange any day in Restore week (Tuesday through Friday). Choose one substitute meal plan and substitute it in for any day you choose.

FOOD ITEM	AVERAGE SERVING SIZE	CALORIES
PROTEIN		
HAMBURGER PATTY	3.5 OZ	235 CAL
TRI TIP	3.5 OZ	182 CAL
PORK CUTLET	3.5 OZ	231 CAL
CHICKEN	4 OZ	190 CAL
BEEF NEW YORK STRIP STEAK	4 OZ	220 CAL
BABY BACK RIBS	3 OZ	270 CAL
PORK SIRLOIN	3 OZ	168 CAL
BEEF RIBEYE STEAK	6 OZ	450 CAL
SALMON	3 OZ	200 CAL
HALIBUT	3 OZ	107 CAL
FRIED EGG	1 LARGE EGG	92 CAL
BOILED EGG	1 LARGE EGG	77 CAL
SCRAMBLED EGG	1 LARGE EGG	101 CAL
CARBOHYDRATES		
BANANA	1 MEDIUM BANANA	104 CAL
APPLE	1 MEDIUM APPLE	80 CAL
ORANGE	1 FRUIT	69 CAL
SPAGHETTI WITH MEAT SAUCE	10 OZ	286 CAL
CHICKEN ALFREDO PASTA	8.14 OZ	321 CAL
WHITE RICE	1 CUP	205 CAL
BROWN RICE	1 CUP	216 CAL
BLACK BEANS	½ CUP	90 CAL
REFRIED BEANS	½ CUP	125 CAL
PINTO BEANS	½ CUP	144 CAL
BROCCOLI	1 CUP	65 CAL
GREEN BEANS	1 CUP	25 CAL
CORN	4 OZ	153 CAL
WHOLE WHEAT BREAD	1 SLICE	69 CAL
WHITE BREAD	1 SLICE	120 CAL
SOURDOUGH BREAD	1 SLICE	120 CAL
RESTAURANTS		
IN N OUT BURGER WITH ONION	1 SERVING	390 CAL

MCDONALDS CHEESEBURGER	1 SERVING	300 CAL
TACO BELL CRUNCHY SUPREME TACO	1 SERVING	190 CAL
TACO BELL BEAN BURRITO	1 SERVING	370 CAL
EL POLLO LOCO AL CARBON CHICKEN TACOS	1 SERVING	160 CAL
JAMBA JUICE ACAI PRIMO FRUIT BOWL	1 SERVING	540 CAL
CARL'S JR SPICY CHICKEN SANDWICH	1 SERVING	460 CAL
SUBWAY HAM SANDWICH 6 INCH	1 SERVING	450 CAL
PANERA BREAD STRAWBERRY POPPYSEED CHICKEN SALAD	1 SERVING	350 CAL
RED LOBSTER STARTER SAMPLER	1 SERVING	620 CAL
OLIVE GARDEN CHICKEN ALFREDO FETTUCCINE	1 SERVING	500 CAL
RED ROBIN WINGS	1 SERVING	1,023 CAL
APPLEBEE'S TRIPLE BACON BURGER	1 SERVING	1,190 CAL

Note: Above is an example of some but not all food items allowed in Combo. Remember you can eat anything you want in Combo (Saturday and Sunday) as long as you stay within your targeted caloric intake.

QUICK START: COMBO	*SATURDAY- SUNDAY: 1,300 CALORIES*
SATURDAY BREAKFAST:	SUNDAY BREAKFAST:
• 2 CUPS HONEY NUT CHEERIOS CEREAL (293 CALORIES) • 1 CUP MILK (108 CALORIES)	• 1 CUP GREEK GODS YOGURT (290 CALORIES) • .5 OZ OATS GRANOLA (95 CALORIES)
SATURDAY LUNCH:	SUNDAY LUNCH:
• SUBWAY SANDWICH (450 CALORIES)	• 4 OZ CORN TORTILLA CHIPS (241 CALORIES) • 10 OZ SALSA (71 CALORIES)
SATURDAY DINNER:	SUNDAY DINNER:
• 1 CUP HORMEL CHILI (260 CALORIES) • 2 OZ CORNBREAD (198 CALORIES)	• 2 CUPS SPAGHETTI (347 CALORIES) • 2 OZ FRENCH BREAD (188 CALORIES)
	SUNDAY SNACK:
	• 1 FAT FREE CHOCOLATE PUDDING CUP (100 CALORIES)
TOTAL: 1,310 CALORIES	TOTAL: 1,333 CALORIES

Note: In Combo you can eat ANY food, but stay in your caloric intake!

Macro Circuit Quick Start

1,500 Calorie Meal Plan

These meal plans are for those people who don't have the time to cook meals and need that quick start.

MONDAY BREAKFAST: (EXAMPLE 1)	MONDAY BREAKFAST: (EXAMPLE 2)
HOT BROTH • 12 OZ BEEF BROTH, HEATED	ORANGE JUICE • 12 OZ ORANGE JUICE (NO PULP)
LUNCH:	LUNCH:
APPLE JUICE • 12 OZ APPLE JUICE	GRAPE JUICE • 12 OZ GRAPE JUICE
DINNER:	DINNER:
CRANBERRY JUICE • 12 OZ CRANBERRY JUICE	TOMATO JUICE • 12 OZ TOMATO JUICE
SNACK:	SNACK:
WATER • 12 OZ WATER	VEGETABLE JUICE • 12 OZ VEGETABLE JUICE

<u>Reminder:</u> These are 2 examples of what your Mondays will look like. DO NOT FOLLOW THIS PLAN.

Things You Can Have During Your Flush: (Calories for 8 fl ounces)

- Coconut Water (46 Calories)
- Water (0 Calories)
- Carrot Juice (94 Calories)
- Apple Juice (105 Calories)
- Orange Juice (115 Calories)
- Grape Juice (152 Calories)
- Vegetable Juice (50 Calories)
- Pomegranate Juice (140 Calories)
- Tomato Juice (41 Calories)
- Grapefruit Juice (102 Calories)
- Cranberry Juice (116 Calories)
- Chicken Broth (41 Calories)
- Beef Broth (10 Calories)
- Tea (nothing added) (2.4 Calories)
- Coffee (nothing added) (1.8 Calories)

Note: This is a 24-hour fast. No food is to be consumed during this time. It is advised to only choose from the options above. Stay within your caloric intake. This meal plan is just an EXAMPLE of what your Mondays should look like.

TUESDAY BREAKFAST:	WEDNESDAY BREAKFAST:

SOUTHWEST SALSA EGGS
- 4 LARGE EGGS
- 3 TBSP SALSA

BANANA, GRAPE, BERRY SMOOTHIE
- ¼ CUP WATER
- ½ MEDIUM BANANA
- ½ CUP BLUEBERRIES
- 1 CUP HALVED STRAWBERRIES
- 20 GRAPES

FRUIT SALAD
- 1 CUP STRAWBERRIES
- 1 CUP BLUEBERRIES

BACON & EGGS
- 2 EGGS
- 2 BACON STRIPS

TUESDAY LUNCH:

WEDNESDAY LUNCH:

CHICKEN
- 6 OZ CHICKEN

DEVILED EGG SALAD
- 4 EXTRA LARGE EGGS
- 2 TBSP MAYONNAISE

TOMATO SOUP
- ½ CAN TOMATO SOUP
- ½ CAN WATER

SLICED RED BELL PEPPER
- 1 MEDIUM RED BELL PEPPER

TUESDAY DINNER:

WEDNESDAY DINNER:

FLANK STEAK
- 6 OZ FLANK STEAK

FILET MIGNON
- 5 OZ BEEF TENDERLOIN

CHERRY TOMATOES
- 1 OZ CHERRY TOMATOES
- 2 CUPS GREEN BEANS

CORN
- 2 SMALL EARS, CORN

TUESDAY SNACK:

WEDNESDAY SNACK:

SPINACH SALAD
- 5 CUPS OF SPINACH
- ½ LEMON YIELDS LEMON JUICE
- 1 TBSP OLIVE OIL

TURKEY & AVOCADO WRAP
- ¼ FRUIT AVOCADO
- 2 OZ DELI CUT TURKEY

BANANA
- 1 MEDIUM BANANA

Thursday and Friday on next page…

THURSDAY BREAKFAST:	FRIDAY BREAKFAST:

THURSDAY BREAKFAST:

EGGS & BACON
- 2 EXTRA LARGE EGGS
- 2 BACON STRIPS

BLUEBERRIES
- 1 CUP BLUEBERRIES
- 1 ORANGE

THURSDAY LUNCH:

QUICK BUFFALO CHICKEN SALAD
- ½ CUP CANNED CHICKEN
- 1 CUP SPINACH
- 1 MEDIUM TOMATO
- 1 CUP CARROTS

THURSDAY DINNER:

SALMON
- 6 OZ ATLANTIC SALMON
- 12 ASPARAGUS SPEARS

THURSDAY SNACK:

CARROT & ORANGE JUICE
- 2 MEDIUM CARROTS
- ½ ORANGE

ALMOND BUTTER & APPLES
- 3 TBSP ALMOND BUTTER
- 2 APPLES

FRIDAY BREAKFAST:

SPINACH, BANANA, CHIA SMOOTHIE
- 1 CUP WATER
- 1 BUNCH SPINACH
- 1 MEDIUM BANANA
- 1 TBSP CHIA SEEDS

EGGS & SAUSAGE OMELETTE
- 6 EGGS
- 3 OZ SAUSAGE

FRIDAY LUNCH:

CHICKEN
- 6 OZ CHICKEN

CARROTS
- 2 LARGE CARROT

FRIDAY DINNER:

TILAPIA
- 6 OZ TILAPIA

BRUSSEL SPROUTS
- 2 CUP BRUSSELS SPROUTS

FRIDAY SNACK:

APPLE & ALMOND BUTTER
- 2 TBSP ALMOND BUTTER AND 1 APPLE

(SUBSTITUTE 1) BREAKFAST:	(SUBSTITUTE 2) BREAKFAST:
MANGO SMOOTHIE	**OVER EASY EGGS**
• 1 FRUIT MANGO	• 4 LARGE EGGS
• 1 CUP COCONUT WATER	
• 1 CUP ICE CUBES	
LUNCH:	
TUNA SALAD	**ORANGES**
• 1 CAN TUNA IN VEGETABLE OIL	• 2 ORANGES
• 2 TBSP MAYONNAISE	
CARROTS & RANCH	
• 1 CUP BABY CARROTS	
• 4 TBSP RANCH DRESSING	
DINNER:	LUNCH:
CHICKEN	**FILET MIGNON**
• 6 OZ GRILLED CHICKEN BREAST	• 4 OZ BEEF TENDERLOIN
	• 1 FL OZ RED WINE
	• 2 TBSP BALSAMIC VINEGAR
BROCCOLI	**CARROTS**
• 4 OZ BROCCOLI	• 1 CUP BABY CARROTS
SNACK:	DINNER:
BANANA & ALMOND BUTTER	**TILAPIA**
• 1 MEDIUM BANANA	• 4 OZ TILAPIA
• 2 TBSP ALMOND BUTTER	• ½ TSP VEGETABLE OIL
	ZUCCHINI
	• 2 MEDIUM ZUCCHINI
	SNACK:
	GRAPES & ALMONDS
	• 2 CUP GRAPES
	• 1 OZ ALMONDS

<u>Note:</u> Above are two full day "substitute" meal plans that can be used to interchange any day in Restore week (Tuesday through Friday). Choose one substitute meal plan and substitute it in for any day you choose.

FOOD ITEM	AVERAGE SERVING SIZE	CALORIES
PROTEIN		
HAMBURGER PATTY	3.5 OZ	235 CAL
TRI TIP	3.5 OZ	182 CAL
PORK CUTLET	3.5 OZ	231 CAL
CHICKEN	4 OZ	190 CAL
BEEF NEW YORK STRIP STEAK	4 OZ	220 CAL
BABY BACK RIBS	3 OZ	270 CAL
PORK SIRLOIN	3 OZ	168 CAL
BEEF RIBEYE STEAK	6 OZ	450 CAL
SALMON	3 OZ	200 CAL
HALIBUT	3 OZ	107 CAL
FRIED EGG	1 LARGE EGG	92 CAL
BOILED EGG	1 LARGE EGG	77 CAL
SCRAMBLED EGG	1 LARGE EGG	101 CAL
CARBOHYDRATES		
BANANA	1 MEDIUM BANANA	104 CAL
APPLE	1 MEDIUM APPLE	80 CAL
ORANGE	1 FRUIT	69 CAL
SPAGHETTI WITH MEAT SAUCE	10 OZ	286 CAL
CHICKEN ALFREDO PASTA	8.14 OZ	321 CAL
WHITE RICE	1 CUP	205 CAL
BROWN RICE	1 CUP	216 CAL
BLACK BEANS	½ CUP	90 CAL
REFRIED BEANS	½ CUP	125 CAL
PINTO BEANS	½ CUP	144 CAL
BROCCOLI	1 CUP	65 CAL
GREEN BEANS	1 CUP	25 CAL
CORN	4 OZ	153 CAL
WHOLE WHEAT BREAD	1 SLICE	69 CAL
WHITE BREAD	1 SLICE	120 CAL
SOURDOUGH BREAD	1 SLICE	120 CAL
RESTAURANTS		
IN N OUT BURGER WITH ONION	1 SERVING	390 CAL

MCDONALDS CHEESEBURGER	1 SERVING	300 CAL
TACO BELL CRUNCHY SUPREME TACO	1 SERVING	190 CAL
TACO BELL BEAN BURRITO	1 SERVING	370 CAL
EL POLLO LOCO AL CARBON CHICKEN TACOS	1 SERVING	160 CAL
JAMBA JUICE ACAI PRIMO FRUIT BOWL	1 SERVING	540 CAL
CARL'S JR SPICY CHICKEN SANDWICH	1 SERVING	460 CAL
SUBWAY HAM SANDWICH 6 INCH	1 SERVING	450 CAL
PANERA BREAD STRAWBERRY POPPYSEED CHICKEN SALAD	1 SERVING	350 CAL
RED LOBSTER STARTER SAMPLER	1 SERVING	620 CAL
OLIVE GARDEN CHICKEN ALFREDO FETTUCCINE	1 SERVING	500 CAL
RED ROBIN WINGS	1 SERVING	1,023 CAL
APPLEBEE'S TRIPLE BACON BURGER	1 SERVING	1,190 CAL

Note: Above is an example of some but not all food items allowed in Combo. Remember you can eat anything you want in Combo (Saturday and Sunday) as long as you stay within your targeted caloric intake.

<table>
<tr><td>

QUICK START: COMBO

</td><td>

SATURDAY- SUNDAY: 1,500 CALORIES

</td></tr>
<tr><td>

SATURDAY BREAKFAST:
- 1 BREAKFAST BURRITO
  (302 CALORIES)

</td><td>

SUNDAY BREAKFAST:
- 2 BUTTERMILK PANCAKES (6" DIA)
  (350 CALORIES)
- 4 TBSP LITE SYRUP
  (105 CALORIES)

</td></tr>
<tr><td>

SATURDAY LUNCH:
- 1 AMIGOS MEXICAN RESTAURANT
  BURRITO
  (500 CALORIES)

</td><td>

SUNDAY LUNCH:
- 2 CRUNCHY TACOS, TACO BELL
  (340 CALORIES)

</td></tr>
<tr><td>

SATURDAY DINNER:
- 1 ENCHILADA
  (323 CALORIES)
- ½ CUP REFRIED BEANS
  (115 CALORIES)

</td><td>

SUNDAY DINNER:
- 6 OZ ORANGE CHICKEN
  (399 CALORIES)

</td></tr>
<tr><td>

SATURDAY SNACK:
- STARBUCKS CARAMEL MACCHIATO
  (190 CALORIES)

</td><td>

SUNDAY SNACK:
- 1 PIECE OF CHEESECAKE
  (257 CALORIES)
- 7 OZ STRAWBERRIES
  (64 CALORIES)

</td></tr>
<tr><td>

TOTAL: 1,429 CALORIES

</td><td>

TOTAL: 1,515 CALORIES

</td></tr>
</table>

<u>Note:</u> In Combo you can eat ANY food, but stay in your caloric intake!

Macro Circuit Quick Start

1,800 Calorie Meal Plan

These meal plans are for those people who don't have the time to cook meals and need that quick start.

MONDAY BREAKFAST: (EXAMPLE 1)	MONDAY BREAKFAST: (EXAMPLE 2)

HOT BROTH
   • 12 OZ BEEF BROTH, HEATED
	ORANGE JUICE
	   • 12 OZ ORANGE JUICE (NO PULP)

LUNCH:	LUNCH:

APPLE JUICE
   • 12 OZ APPLE JUICE
	GRAPE JUICE
	   • 12 OZ GRAPE JUICE

DINNER:	DINNER:

CRANBERRY JUICE
   • 12 OZ CRANBERRY JUICE
	TOMATO JUICE
	   • 12 OZ TOMATO JUICE

SNACK:	SNACK:

WATER
   • 12 OZ WATER
	VEGETABLE JUICE
	   • 12 OZ VEGETABLE JUICE

<u>Reminder:</u> These are 2 examples of what your Mondays will look like. DO NOT FOLLOW THIS PLAN.

Things You Can Have During Your Flush: (Calories for 8 fl ounces)

- Coconut Water (46 Calories)
- Water (0 Calories)
- Carrot Juice (94 Calories)
- Apple Juice (105 Calories)
- Orange Juice (115 Calories)
- Grape Juice (152 Calories)
- Vegetable Juice (50 Calories)
- Pomegranate Juice (140 Calories)
- Tomato Juice (41 Calories)
- Grapefruit Juice (102 Calories)
- Cranberry Juice (116 Calories)
- Chicken Broth (41 Calories)
- Beef Broth (10 Calories)
- Tea (nothing added) (2.4 Calories)
- Coffee (nothing added) (1.8 Calories)

Note: This is a 24-hour fast. No food is to be consumed during this time. It is advised to only choose from the options above. Stay within your caloric intake. This meal plan is just an EXAMPLE of what your Mondays should look like.

TUESDAY BREAKFAST:

OMELET
- 2 EXTRA LARGE EGGS
- 2 SLICES HAM
- 1 TBSP OLIVE OIL

TUESDAY LUNCH:

OSTRICH FILLET
- 8 OZ OSTRICH STEAK
- 2 TBSP OLIVE OIL

CARROTS
- 1 CUP BABY CARROTS

TUESDAY DINNER:

CHICKEN BREAST
- 4 OZ CHICKEN BREAST
- ¼ TSP OLIVE OIL

GRAPES
- 3 CUPS GRAPES

TUESDAY SNACK:

APPLE AND ALMOND BUTTER
- 2 APPLES
- 4 TSP ALMOND BUTTER

WEDNESDAY BREAKFAST:

EGG WHITE, AVOCADO, TOMATO SCRAMBLE
- 4 EGG WHITES
- 2 EGGS
- 1 MEDIUM TOMATO
- ½ FRUIT AVOCADO
- 1 TSP SRIRACHA

STRAWBERRIES
- 2 CUPS STRAWBERRIES

WEDNESDAY LUNCH:

QUICK SALMON
- 8 OZ ATLANTIC SALMON
- ½ TBSP OLIVE OIL

BROCCOLI
- 6 OZ BROCCOLI
- ¼ TBSP OLIVE OIL

WEDNESDAY DINNER:

BARBECUE CHICKEN & LEMON STEAMED BROCCOLI
- 8 OZ CHICKEN
- 4 TBSP BARBECUE SAUCE
- 2 TBSP OLIVE OIL
- 6 OZ BROCCOLI
- 1 TSP LEMON JUICE

WEDNESDAY SNACK:

BANANA
- 2 MEDIUM BANANAS

Thursday and Friday on next page…

QUICK START: RESTORE

THURSDAY BREAKFAST:

QUICK BREAKFAST

- 3 STRIPS BACON
- 1 MEDIUM BANANA

THURSDAY LUNCH:

HONEY GLAZED SALTED SALMON

- 12 OZ PINK SALMON
- 1 ½ TBSP HONEY
- 2 EARS OF CORN

THURSDAY DINNER:

BAKED BARBECUE CHICKEN

- 4 OZ CHICKEN BREAST
- 2 TBSP BARBECUE SAUCE
- 1 TBSP OLIVE OIL

THURSDAY SNACK:

TURKEY LETTUCE ROLL UP

- 6 OUTER LETTUCE LEAVES
- 6 SLICES DELI TURKEY

CELERY

- 4 STALKS CELERY

THURSDAY - FRIDAY: 1,800 CALORIES

FRIDAY BREAKFAST:

SIMPLE SPINACH SCRAMBLE

- 4 TSP OLIVE OIL
- 2 CUPS SPINACH
- 4 LARGE EGGS

FRIDAY LUNCH:

EASY GRILLED CHICKEN & CORN

- 6 OZ CHICKEN BREAST
- 1 SMALL EAR, CORN

ROASTED ASPARAGUS

- 6 ASPARAGUS SPEARS
- 1 TBSP OLIVE OIL

FRIDAY DINNER:

SIMPLE STEAK AND CARROTS

- 1 BEEF STEAK (136 G)
- 3 CUPS CARROTS

FRIDAY SNACK:

APPLE AND ALMOND BUTTER

- 1 MEDIUM APPLE
- 2 TBSP ALMOND BUTTER

(SUBSTITUTE 1) BREAKFAST:	(SUBSTITUTE 2) BREAKFAST:

SAUSAGE AND EGG WHITE SCRAMBLE

- 1 ½ CUP EGG WHITES
- 1 EGG
- 2 TBSP OLIVE OIL
- 2 OZ SAUSAGE

SCRAMBLED EGGS WITH MUSHROOMS

- 2 TBSP OLIVE OIL
- 2 CUP WHOLE MUSHROOM
- 4 LARGE EGGS
- 2 MEDIUM ONIONS

APPLE

- 2 APPLES

APPLE

- 1 APPLE

LUNCH:

MANGO STRAWBERRY SALAD

- 1 MANGO WITHOUT REFUSE
- 5 MEDIUM STRAWBERRIES
- 3 TBSP ORANGE JUICE
- 2 TSP HONEY

SLICE IT UP. MIX IT. SERVE.

DINNER:

LUNCH:

GRILLED CHICKEN MEDITERRANEAN

- 8 OZ CHICKEN BREAST
- 3/4 TBSP OLIVE OIL
- ¼ CUP CHERRY TOMATOES
- ¼ CUP OLIVES

CHICKEN

- 8 OZ CHICKEN BREAST
- 2 TSP OLIVE OIL

TOMATO SOUP

- ½ CAN TOMATO SOUP
- ½ CUP WATER

MIX. HEAT. SERVE.

DINNER:

BROCCOLI

- 6 OZ BROCCOLI

FILET MIGNON

- 4 OZ BEEF TENDERLOIN
- 1 FL OZ RED WINE
- 1 OZ BALSAMIC VINEGAR

SNACK:

TURKEY LETTUCE ROLL UP

- 6 OUTER LETTUCE LEAVES
- 6 SLICES DELI TURKEY

STEAMED BROCCOLI

- 6 OZ BROCCOLI
- 2 TSP OLIVE OIL

SNACK:

BANANA AND ALMOND BUTTER

- 1 MEDIUM BANANA
- 1 TBSP ALMOND BUTTER

CELERY

- 2 STALK, MEDIUM CELERY

<u>Note:</u> Above are two full day "substitute" meal plans that can be used to interchange any day in Restore week (Tuesday through Friday). Choose one substitute meal plan and substitute it in for any day you choose.

FOOD ITEM	AVERAGE SERVING SIZE	CALORIES
PROTEIN		
HAMBURGER PATTY	3.5 OZ	235 CAL
TRI TIP	3.5 OZ	182 CAL
PORK CUTLET	3.5 OZ	231 CAL
CHICKEN	4 OZ	190 CAL
BEEF NEW YORK STRIP STEAK	4 OZ	220 CAL
BABY BACK RIBS	3 OZ	270 CAL
PORK SIRLOIN	3 OZ	168 CAL
BEEF RIBEYE STEAK	6 OZ	450 CAL
SALMON	3 OZ	200 CAL
HALIBUT	3 OZ	107 CAL
FRIED EGG	1 LARGE EGG	92 CAL
BOILED EGG	1 LARGE EGG	77 CAL
SCRAMBLED EGG	1 LARGE EGG	101 CAL
CARBOHYDRATES		
BANANA	1 MEDIUM BANANA	104 CAL
APPLE	1 MEDIUM APPLE	80 CAL
ORANGE	1 FRUIT	69 CAL
SPAGHETTI WITH MEAT SAUCE	10 OZ	286 CAL
CHICKEN ALFREDO PASTA	8.14 OZ	321 CAL
WHITE RICE	1 CUP	205 CAL
BROWN RICE	1 CUP	216 CAL
BLACK BEANS	½ CUP	90 CAL
REFRIED BEANS	½ CUP	125 CAL
PINTO BEANS	½ CUP	144 CAL
BROCCOLI	1 CUP	65 CAL
GREEN BEANS	1 CUP	25 CAL
CORN	4 OZ	153 CAL
WHOLE WHEAT BREAD	1 SLICE	69 CAL
WHITE BREAD	1 SLICE	120 CAL
SOURDOUGH BREAD	1 SLICE	120 CAL
RESTAURANTS		
IN N OUT BURGER WITH ONION	1 SERVING	390 CAL

MCDONALDS CHEESEBURGER	1 SERVING	300 CAL
TACO BELL CRUNCHY SUPREME TACO	1 SERVING	190 CAL
TACO BELL BEAN BURRITO	1 SERVING	370 CAL
EL POLLO LOCO AL CARBON CHICKEN TACOS	1 SERVING	160 CAL
JAMBA JUICE ACAI PRIMO FRUIT BOWL	1 SERVING	540 CAL
CARL'S JR SPICY CHICKEN SANDWICH	1 SERVING	460 CAL
SUBWAY HAM SANDWICH 6 INCH	1 SERVING	450 CAL
PANERA BREAD STRAWBERRY POPPYSEED CHICKEN SALAD	1 SERVING	350 CAL
RED LOBSTER STARTER SAMPLER	1 SERVING	620 CAL
OLIVE GARDEN CHICKEN ALFREDO FETTUCCINE	1 SERVING	500 CAL
RED ROBIN WINGS	1 SERVING	1,023 CAL
APPLEBEE'S TRIPLE BACON BURGER	1 SERVING	1,190 CAL

Note: Above is an example of some but not all food items allowed in Combo. Remember you can eat anything you want in Combo (Saturday and Sunday) as long as you stay within your targeted caloric intake.

QUICK START: COMBO   *SATURDAY- SUNDAY: 1,800 CALORIES*

SATURDAY BREAKFAST:
- 3 WAFFLES
  (278 CALORIES)
- 2 EGGS
  (140 CALORIES)
- 4 TBSP LITE SYRUP
  (105 CALORIES)

SATURDAY LUNCH:
- 1 PANERA GRILLED CHICKEN CAESAR SALAD
  (400 CALORIES)
- 4 TBSP HIDDEN VALLEY RANCH DRESSING
  (220 CALORIES)

SATURDAY DINNER:
- 4 OZ TRI TIP
  (171 CALORIES)
- 1 BAKED POTATO
  (145 CALORIES)
- 1 CUP MIXED VEGGIES
  (20 CALORIES)

SATURDAY SNACK:
- JAMBA JUICE STRAWBERRY WILD
  (370 CALORIES)

TOTAL: 1,849 CALORIES

SUNDAY BREAKFAST:
- 2 EGGS
  (140 CALORIES)
- 1 CUP HASHBROWN POTATOES
  (413 CALORIES)
- 1 OZ PORK CHORIZO
  (49 CALORIES)

SUNDAY LUNCH:
- 1 IN N OUT HAMBURGER (390 CALORIES)
- 1 SMALL FRY
  (230 CALORIES)

SUNDAY DINNER:
- 1 CUP MEATLOAF
  (660 CALORIES)

TOTAL: 1,882 CALORIES

<u>Note:</u> In Combo you can eat ANY food, but stay in your caloric intake!

Macro Circuit Quick Start

2,000 Calorie Meal Plan

These meal plans are for those people who don't have the time to cook meals and need that quick start.

QUICK START: FLUSH	*MONDAY: 2,000 CALORIES*
MONDAY BREAKFAST: (EXAMPLE 1)	MONDAY BREAKFAST: (EXAMPLE 2)

HOT BROTH
   •   12 OZ BEEF BROTH, HEATED
	ORANGE JUICE
	   • 12 OZ ORANGE JUICE (NO PULP)

LUNCH:
APPLE JUICE
   •   12 OZ APPLE JUICE
	LUNCH:
	GRAPE JUICE
	   • 12 OZ GRAPE JUICE

DINNER:
CRANBERRY JUICE
   •   12 OZ CRANBERRY JUICE
	DINNER:
	TOMATO JUICE
	   • 12 OZ TOMATO JUICE

SNACK:
WATER
   •   12 OZ WATER
	SNACK:
	VEGETABLE JUICE
	   • 12 OZ VEGETABLE JUICE

<u>Reminder:</u> These are 2 examples of what your Mondays will look like. DO NOT FOLLOW THIS PLAN.

Things You Can Have During Your Flush: (Calories for 8 fl ounces)

- Coconut Water (46 Calories)
- Water (0 Calories)
- Carrot Juice (94 Calories)
- Apple Juice (105 Calories)
- Orange Juice (115 Calories)
- Grape Juice (152 Calories)
- Vegetable Juice (50 Calories)
- Pomegranate Juice (140 Calories)
- Tomato Juice (41 Calories)
- Grapefruit Juice (102 Calories)
- Cranberry Juice (116 Calories)
- Chicken Broth (41 Calories)
- Beef Broth (10 Calories)
- Tea (nothing added) (2.4 Calories)
- Coffee (nothing added) (1.8 Calories)

Note: This is a 24-hour fast. No food is to be consumed during this time. It is advised to only choose from the options above. Stay within your caloric intake. This meal plan is just an EXAMPLE of what your Mondays should look like.

TUESDAY BREAKFAST:	**WEDNESDAY BREAKFAST:**

SIMPLE SPINACH SCRAMBLE
- 1 CUP SPINACH
- 3 LARGE EGGS

SAUSAGE AND EGG
- ¾ CUP EGG WHITES
- 2 OZ SAUSAGE
- 2 EGGS

TUESDAY LUNCH:

BARBECUE CHICKEN
- 6 OZ CHICKEN
- 3 TBSP BARBECUE SAUCE

APPLES
- 3 APPLES

WEDNESDAY LUNCH:

CARROTS & ASPARAGUS
- 3 CUPS BABY CARROTS
- 12 SPEARS, ASPARAGUS

FILET MIGNON WITH RICH BALSAMIC GLAZE
- 4 OZ BEEF TENDERLOIN
- 2 TBSP BALSAMIC VINEGAR
- 1 FL OZ RED WINE

TUESDAY DINNER:

BAKED TILAPIA
- 14 OZ TILAPIA
- 1 TBSP OLIVE OIL

BANANA
- 1 MEDIUM BANANA

TUESDAY SNACKS:

BANANA AND ALMOND BUTTER
- 1 MEDIUM BANANA
- 1 TBSP ALMOND BUTTER

WEDNESDAY DINNER:

BAKED BARBECUE CHICKEN
- 4 OZ CHICKEN
- 2 TBSP BARBECUE SAUCE
- 1 TBSP OLIVE OIL

CARROTS
- 2 CUPS BABY CARROTS

CARROTS
- 1 CUP BABY CARROTS

WEDNESDAY SNACK:

ALMONDS
- 1 OZ ALMONDS

TUNA SALAD
- 1 CAN TUNA
- 1 TBSP LEMON JUICE

CELERY AND ALMOND BUTTER
- 4 TBSP ALMOND BUTTER
- 4 STALKS CELERY

Thursday and Friday on next page…

QUICK START: RESTORE	*TUESDAY-WEDNESDAY: 2,000 CALORIES*

THURSDAY BREAKFAST:
BANANA, ORANGE, GRAPE SHAKE
- ½ MEDIUM BANANA
- ½ CUP ORANGE JUICE
- ¼ CUP GRAPES

THURSDAY LUNCH:

CHICKEN BREAST
- 6 OZ BREAST CHICKEN
- 1 TBSP OLIVE OIL

BROCCOLI
- 3 CUPS BROCCOLI
- 1 TBSP OLIVE OIL

BANANA
- 1 BANANA

THURSDAY DINNER:
HONEY SALMON
- 6 OZ PINK SALMON
- ½ TSP HONEY
- ½ TBSP CANOLA OIL

ZUCCHINI
- 2 MEDIUM ZUCCHINI

AVOCADO
- 1 FRUIT AVOCADO

THURSDAY SNACK:
BANANA AND ALMOND BUTTER
- 1 MEDIUM BANANA
- 1 TBSP ALMOND BUTTER

CARROTS
- 1 CUP BABY CARROTS

FRIDAY BREAKFAST:
EGGS
- 4 LARGE EGGS
- 1 TBSP OLIVE OIL

BACON
- 3 STRIPS BACON

FRIDAY LUNCH:

CHICKEN BREAST
- 6 OZ CHICKEN BREAST

BROCCOLI
- 3 CUPS BROCCOLI
- 1 TBSP OLIVE OIL

FRIDAY DINNER:
STEAK & ASPARAGUS
- 8 OZ FLANK STEAK
- 2 CUPS ASPARAGUS

FRIDAY SNACK:
TURKEY LETTUCE WRAP
- 6 OUTER LETTUCE LEAVES
- 6 SLICES DELI TURKEY

ALMONDS
- 2 OZ ALMONDS

BANANA
- 1 MEDIUM BANANA

(SUBSTITUTE 1) BREAKFAST:

PESTO EGG SCRAMBLE
- 1 TBSP OLIVE OIL
- 4 LARGE EGGS
- ½ TBSP BASIL PESTO

LUNCH:

CHICKEN
- 6 OZ CHICKEN BREAST
- ¾ CUP ITALIAN DRESSING

ASPARAGUS
- 2 CUPS ASPARAGUS
- ¼ TBSP OLIVE OIL

DINNER:

CHICKEN BREAST
- 6 OZ CHICKEN BREAST
- ½ TSP OLIVE OIL

CORN EAR
- 2 EARS OF CORN
- 1 TBSP BUTTER

SNACK:

GRAPES
- 2 CUPS GRAPES

CELERY AND ALMOND BUTTER
- 2 TBSP ALMOND BUTTER
- 2 STALKS CELERY

(SUBSTITUTE 2) BREAKFAST:

EGGS
- 4 LARGE EGGS

BACON
- 2 STRIPS BACON

CANTALOUPE
- 6 WEDGES OF CANTALOUPE

LUNCH:

BEEF
- 8 OZ BEEF TENDERLOIN

ZUCCHINI
- 2 MEDIUM ZUCCHINI

DINNER:

BARBECUE CHICKEN
- 4 OZ CHICKEN BREAST
- 2 TBSP BARBECUE SAUCE
- 1 TBSP OLIVE OIL

CARROTS
- 3 CUPS BABY CARROTS

SNACK:

ALMOND BUTTER AND CELERY
- 2 TBSP ALMOND BUTTER
- 2 STALKS CELERY

<u>Note</u>: Above are two full day "substitute" meal plans that can be used to interchange any day in Restore week (Tuesday through Friday). Choose one substitute meal plan and substitute it in for any day you choose.

FOOD ITEM	AVERAGE SERVING SIZE	CALORIES
PROTEIN		
HAMBURGER PATTY	3.5 OZ	235 CAL
TRI TIP	3.5 OZ	182 CAL
PORK CUTLET	3.5 OZ	231 CAL
CHICKEN	4 OZ	190 CAL
BEEF NEW YORK STRIP STEAK	4 OZ	220 CAL
BABY BACK RIBS	3 OZ	270 CAL
PORK SIRLOIN	3 OZ	168 CAL
BEEF RIBEYE STEAK	6 OZ	450 CAL
SALMON	3 OZ	200 CAL
HALIBUT	3 OZ	107 CAL
FRIED EGG	1 LARGE EGG	92 CAL
BOILED EGG	1 LARGE EGG	77 CAL
SCRAMBLED EGG	1 LARGE EGG	101 CAL
CARBOHYDRATES		
BANANA	1 MEDIUM BANANA	104 CAL
APPLE	1 MEDIUM APPLE	80 CAL
ORANGE	1 FRUIT	69 CAL
SPAGHETTI WITH MEAT SAUCE	10 OZ	286 CAL
CHICKEN ALFREDO PASTA	8.14 OZ	321 CAL
WHITE RICE	1 CUP	205 CAL
BROWN RICE	1 CUP	216 CAL
BLACK BEANS	½ CUP	90 CAL
REFRIED BEANS	½ CUP	125 CAL
PINTO BEANS	½ CUP	144 CAL
BROCCOLI	1 CUP	65 CAL
GREEN BEANS	1 CUP	25 CAL
CORN	4 OZ	153 CAL
WHOLE WHEAT BREAD	1 SLICE	69 CAL
WHITE BREAD	1 SLICE	120 CAL
SOURDOUGH BREAD	1 SLICE	120 CAL
RESTAURANTS		
IN N OUT BURGER WITH ONION	1 SERVING	390 CAL

MCDONALDS CHEESEBURGER	1 SERVING	300 CAL
TACO BELL CRUNCHY SUPREME TACO	1 SERVING	190 CAL
TACO BELL BEAN BURRITO	1 SERVING	370 CAL
EL POLLO LOCO AL CARBON CHICKEN TACOS	1 SERVING	160 CAL
JAMBA JUICE ACAI PRIMO FRUIT BOWL	1 SERVING	540 CAL
CARL'S JR SPICY CHICKEN SANDWICH	1 SERVING	460 CAL
SUBWAY HAM SANDWICH 6 INCH	1 SERVING	450 CAL
PANERA BREAD STRAWBERRY POPPYSEED CHICKEN SALAD	1 SERVING	350 CAL
RED LOBSTER STARTER SAMPLER	1 SERVING	620 CAL
OLIVE GARDEN CHICKEN ALFREDO FETTUCCINE	1 SERVING	500 CAL
RED ROBIN WINGS	1 SERVING	1,023 CAL
APPLEBEE'S TRIPLE BACON BURGER	1 SERVING	1,190 CAL

Note: Above is an example of some but not all food items allowed in Combo. Remember you can eat anything you want in Combo (Saturday and Sunday) as long as you stay within your targeted caloric intake.

QUICK START: COMBO	*SATURDAY- SUNDAY: 2,000 CALORIES*

SATURDAY BREAKFAST:

- 2 IHOP EGGS (140 CALORIES)
- 1 SERVING IHOP HASH BROWNS (224 CALORIES)
- 1 IHOP BACON (40 CALORIES)
- 1 IHOP PANCAKE (157 CALORIES)
- .5 OZ IHOP SYRUP (55 CALORIES)

SATURDAY LUNCH:

- TUNA MELT (408 CALORIES)
- 1 CHEETO SNACK BAG (160 CALORIES)

SATURDAY DINNER:

- 1 PERSONAL PIZZA (850 CALORIES)

SATURDAY SNACK:

- JAMBA JUICE STRAWBERRY WILD (370 CALORIES)

TOTAL: 2,033 CALORIES

SUNDAY BREAKFAST:

- 1.5 CUPS LUCKY CHARMS CEREAL (220 CALORIES)
- 1 CUP MILK (108 CALORIES)

SUNDAY LUNCH:

- 10 BBQ WINGS (880 CALORIES)
- 8 FL OZ SODA (119 CALORIES)

SUNDAY DINNER:

- 4 OZ CHICKEN (253 CALORIES)
- 1 CUP SUPER SWEET CORN (120 CALORIES)
- 1 BEER (306 CALORIES)

TOTAL: 2,007 CALORIES

<u>Note:</u> In Combo you can eat ANY food, but stay in your caloric intake!

Macro Circuit Quick Start

2,500 Calorie Meal Plan

These meal plans are for those people who don't have the time to cook meals and need that quick start.

MONDAY BREAKFAST: (EXAMPLE 1)	MONDAY BREAKFAST: (EXAMPLE 2)
HOT BROTH	ORANGE JUICE
• 12 OZ BEEF BROTH, HEATED	• 12 OZ ORANGE JUICE (NO PULP)
LUNCH:	LUNCH:
APPLE JUICE	GRAPE JUICE
• 12 OZ APPLE JUICE	• 12 OZ GRAPEFRUIT
DINNER:	DINNER:
CRANBERRY JUICE	TOMATO JUICE
• 12 OZ CRANBERRY JUICE	• 12 OZ TOMATO JUICE
SNACK:	SNACK:
WATER	VEGETABLE JUICE
• 12 OZ WATER	• 12 OZ VEGETABLE JUICE

<u>Reminder:</u> These are 2 examples of what your Mondays will look like. DO NOT FOLLOW THIS PLAN.

Things You Can Have During Your Flush: (Calories for 8 fl ounces)

- Coconut Water (46 Calories)
- Water (0 Calories)
- Carrot Juice (94 Calories)
- Apple Juice (105 Calories)
- Orange Juice (115 Calories)
- Grape Juice (152 Calories)
- Vegetable Juice (50 Calories)
- Pomegranate Juice (140 Calories)
- Tomato Juice (41 Calories)
- Grapefruit Juice (102 Calories)
- Cranberry Juice (116 Calories)
- Chicken Broth (41 Calories)
- Beef Broth (10 Calories)
- Tea (nothing added) (2.4 Calories)
- Coffee (nothing added) (1.8 Calories)

Note: This is a 24-hour fast. No food is to be consumed during this time. It is advised to only choose from the options above. Stay within your caloric intake. This meal plan is just an EXAMPLE of what your Mondays should look like.

TUESDAY BREAKFAST:

EGGS & ORANGES

- 4 EGGS
- 1TBSP VEGETABLE OIL
- 2 ORANGES

BACON

- 3 STRIPS BACON

TUESDAY LUNCH:

CHICKEN & GREEN BEANS

- 10 OZ CHICKEN BREAST
- 2 CUPS GREEN BEANS

TUESDAY DINNER:

STEAK & ASPARAGUS

- 8 OZ SIRLOIN STEAK
- 12 SPEARS

CARROTS

- 2 CUPS BABY CARROTS

TUESDAY SNACK:

LEMON PEPPER TUNA

- 1 CAN TUNA, CANNED IN WATER
- ½ TSP PEPPER
- 1 TBSP LEMON JUICE

BANANAS

- 2 MEDIUM BANANAS

WEDNESDAY BREAKFAST:

SPINACH SCRAMBLED EGGS

- 4 EXTRA LARGE EGGS
- 2 CUPS SPINACH
- 2 TBSP OLIVE OIL

WEDNESDAY LUNCH:

GRILLED SCALLOPS

- 18 OZ SCALLOPS
- 1 TBSP OLIVE OIL

ALMONDS

- 1 OZ ALMONDS

WEDNESDAY DINNER:

STEAK

- 8 OZ BEEF STEAK
- 2 TBSP OLIVE OIL

ASPARAGUS

- 8 OZ ASPARAGUS
- ½ TBSP OLIVE OIL

WEDNESDAY SNACK:

GRAPES

- 3 CUPS GRAPES

CARROTS

- 1 CUP BABY CARROTS

Thursday and Friday on next page…

QUICK START: RESTORE	*THURSDAY- FRIDAY: 2,500 CALORIES*

THURSDAY BREAKFAST:

6 BANANA EGG PANCAKES

- 3 MEDIUM BANANAS
- 6 LARGE EGGS
- BLEND. COOK.

ORANGES

- 3 FRUIT ORANGES

THURSDAY LUNCH:

BASIC ROAST BEEF

- 10 OZ BEEF CHUNK
- 1 TSP OLIVE OIL

TOSSED SALAD

- 1 CUP SHREDDED LETTUCE
- 1 TBSP RANCH DRESSING
- 1 CUCUMBER
- 1 LARGE CARROT
- 1 MEDIUM TOMATO

THURSDAY DINNER:

BAKED CHICKEN

- 5 OZ CHICKEN BREAST
- .5 OZ UNSALTED BUTTER

PAN FRIED CORN

- 1 LARGE EAR OF CORN
- 1 TBSP BUTTER

THURSDAY SNACK:

BANANA

- 1 MEDIUM BANANA

CARROTS

- 1 CUP BABY CARROTS

FRIDAY BREAKFAST:

6 BANANA EGG PANCAKES

- 3 MEDIUM BANANAS
- 6 LARGE EGGS
- BLEND. COOK.

ORANGES

- 2 FRUIT ORANGES

FRIDAY LUNCH:

ROASTED SALMON

- 5 OZ ATLANTIC SALMON
- 1 TSP OLIVE OIL

SAUTEED GREEN BEANS

- ½ TSP OLIVE OIL
- 3 OZ GREEN BEANS

FRIDAY DINNER:

CHICKEN AND VEGGIES

- 12 OZ CHICKEN BREAST
- ¾ CUPS ITALIAN DRESSING
- 8 OZ RED BELL PEPPERS
- 8 OZ ZUCCHINI

BRUSSEL SPROUTS

- 4 OZ BRUSSELS SPROUTS
- 1 TSP OLIVE OIL

FRIDAY SNACK:

ALMOND BUTTER AND CELERY

- 4 TBSP ALMOND BUTTER
- 4 STALKS LARGE CELERY

PLAIN POPCORN

- .6 OZ POPCORN
- ½ TBSP VEGETABLE OIL

(SUBSTITUTE 1) BREAKFAST:	(SUBSTITUTE 2) BREAKFAST:
SAUSAGE AND EGG WHITE SCRAMBLE • ¾ CUP EGG WHITES • 2 OZ SAUSAGE	**KALE AND EGG** • 2 TSP OLIVE OIL • 2 CUPS KALE • 4 EXTRA LARGE EGGS
APPLE • 1 APPLE	**PECANS** • 1 OZ PECANS

LUNCH:	LUNCH:
FILET MIGNON WITH RICH BALSAMIC GLAZE • 8 OZ BEEF TENDERLOIN • ¼ CUP BALSAMIC VINEGAR • 2 FL OZ RED WINE	**TILAPIA** • 4 OZ TILAPIA • 1 TSP VEGETABLE OIL • 1 TBSP MAPLE SYRUP • 1 TBSP HOISIN SAUCE • 1 TSP DIJON MUSTARD
BRUSSEL SPROUTS • 2 CUPS BRUSSELS SPROUTS • 2 TBSP COCONUT OIL	**BROCCOLI** • 2 CUPS BROCCOLI • 2 TBSP OLIVE OIL

DINNER:	DINNER:
PEACHY KEEN CHICKEN • 1 ½ CUP PEACHES, HALVES • 12 OZ CHICKEN BREAST • 2 TSP HONEY • 2 TSP OLIVE OIL	**GRILLED STEAK WITH PEPPERS** • 10 OZ SIRLOIN STEAK • 1 TSP OLIVE OIL • 1 TBSP BALSAMIC VINEGAR • ½ ONION • 1 CUP RED BELL PEPPERS
ALMONDS • 2 OZ ALMONDS	**ZUCCHINI** • 2 MEDIUM ZUCCHINIS

SNACK:	SNACK:
GRAPES • 1 CUP GRAPES	**GRAPES** • 3 CUPS GRAPES
CARROTS • 3 CUPS BABY CARROTS	

<u>Note:</u> Above are two full day "substitute" meal plans that can be used to interchange any day in Restore week (Tuesday through Friday). Choose one substitute meal plan and substitute it in for any day you choose.

FOOD ITEM	AVERAGE SERVING SIZE	CALORIES
PROTEIN		
HAMBURGER PATTY	3.5 OZ	235 CAL
TRI TIP	3.5 OZ	182 CAL
PORK CUTLET	3.5 OZ	231 CAL
CHICKEN	4 OZ	190 CAL
BEEF NEW YORK STRIP STEAK	4 OZ	220 CAL
BABY BACK RIBS	3 OZ	270 CAL
PORK SIRLOIN	3 OZ	168 CAL
BEEF RIBEYE STEAK	6 OZ	450 CAL
SALMON	3 OZ	200 CAL
HALIBUT	3 OZ	107 CAL
FRIED EGG	1 LARGE EGG	92 CAL
BOILED EGG	1 LARGE EGG	77 CAL
SCRAMBLED EGG	1 LARGE EGG	101 CAL
CARBOHYDRATES		
BANANA	1 MEDIUM BANANA	104 CAL
APPLE	1 MEDIUM APPLE	80 CAL
ORANGE	1 FRUIT	69 CAL
SPAGHETTI WITH MEAT SAUCE	10 OZ	286 CAL
CHICKEN ALFREDO PASTA	8.14 OZ	321 CAL
WHITE RICE	1 CUP	205 CAL
BROWN RICE	1 CUP	216 CAL
BLACK BEANS	½ CUP	90 CAL
REFRIED BEANS	½ CUP	125 CAL
PINTO BEANS	½ CUP	144 CAL
BROCCOLI	1 CUP	65 CAL
GREEN BEANS	1 CUP	25 CAL
CORN	4 OZ	153 CAL
WHOLE WHEAT BREAD	1 SLICE	69 CAL
WHITE BREAD	1 SLICE	120 CAL
SOURDOUGH BREAD	1 SLICE	120 CAL
RESTAURANTS		
IN N OUT BURGER WITH ONION	1 SERVING	390 CAL

MCDONALDS CHEESEBURGER	1 SERVING	300 CAL
TACO BELL CRUNCHY SUPREME TACO	1 SERVING	190 CAL
TACO BELL BEAN BURRITO	1 SERVING	370 CAL
EL POLLO LOCO AL CARBON CHICKEN TACOS	1 SERVING	160 CAL
JAMBA JUICE ACAI PRIMO FRUIT BOWL	1 SERVING	540 CAL
CARL'S JR SPICY CHICKEN SANDWICH	1 SERVING	460 CAL
SUBWAY HAM SANDWICH 6 INCH	1 SERVING	450 CAL
PANERA BREAD STRAWBERRY POPPYSEED CHICKEN SALAD	1 SERVING	350 CAL
RED LOBSTER STARTER SAMPLER	1 SERVING	620 CAL
OLIVE GARDEN CHICKEN ALFREDO FETTUCCINE	1 SERVING	500 CAL
RED ROBIN WINGS	1 SERVING	1,023 CAL
APPLEBEE'S TRIPLE BACON BURGER	1 SERVING	1,190 CAL

Note: Above is an example of some but not all food items allowed in Combo. Remember you can eat anything you want in Combo (Saturday and Sunday) as long as you stay within your targeted caloric intake.

QUICK START: COMBO

SATURDAY- SUNDAY: 2,500 CALORIES

SATURDAY BREAKFAST:	SUNDAY BREAKFAST:

- 2 CHOCOLATE DONUTS (740 CALORIES)
- CARAMEL MACCHIATO COFFEE (190 CALORIES)

— SUNDAY BREAKFAST:

- 1 SERVING BREAKFAST BURRITO (700 CALORIES)

SATURDAY LUNCH:

- 1 JIMMY JOHN BLT (441 CALORIES)
- 1 BAKED LAYS CHIP SNACK BAG (100 CALORIES)
- 8 FL OZ SODA (119 CALORIES)

SUNDAY LUNCH:

- 6 TACOS AL CARBON, EL POLLO LOCO (960 CALORIES)

SATURDAY DINNER:

- 1 SERVING PASTA FETTUCCINE ALFREDO, OLIVE GARDEN (500 CALORIES)
- 2 BREAD STICKS, OLIVE GARDEN (300 CALORIES)
- 8 FL OZ PINK LEMONADE (100 CALORIES)

SUNDAY DINNER:

- 3 CUPS CHICKEN AND VEGGIE STIR FRY (690 CALORIES)
- 1 BEER (153 CALORIES)

TOTAL: 2,490 CALORIES   TOTAL: 2,503 CALORIES

<u>Note:</u> In Combo you can eat ANY food, but stay in your caloric intake!

Macro Circuit Recipe

1,000 Calorie Meal Plan

These meal plans are for those people who have the extra time to cook meals with recipes.

RECIPE: FLUSH   *MONDAY: 1,000 CALORIES*

MONDAY BREAKFAST: (EXAMPLE 1)	MONDAY BREAKFAST: (EXAMPLE 2)
HOT BROTH	ORANGE JUICE
• 12 OZ BEEF BROTH, HEATED	• 12 OZ ORANGE JUICE (NO PULP)
LUNCH:	LUNCH:
APPLE JUICE	GRAPE JUICE
• 12 OZ APPLE JUICE	• 12 OZ GRAPEFRUIT
DINNER:	DINNER:
CRANBERRY JUICE	TOMATO JUICE
• 12 OZ CRANBERRY JUICE	• 12 OZ TOMATO JUICE
SNACK:	SNACK:
WATER	VEGETABLE JUICE
• 12 OZ WATER	• 12 OZ VEGETABLE JUICE

<u>Reminder:</u> These are 2 examples of what your Mondays will look like. DO NOT FOLLOW THIS PLAN.

Things You Can Have During Your Flush: (Calories for 8 fl ounces)

- Coconut Water (46 Calories)

- Water (0 Calories)

- Carrot Juice (94 Calories)

- Apple Juice (105 Calories)

- Orange Juice (115 Calories)

- Grape Juice (152 Calories)

- Vegetable Juice (50 Calories)

- Pomegranate Juice (140 Calories)

- Tomato Juice (41 Calories)

- Grapefruit Juice (102 Calories)

- Cranberry Juice (116 Calories)

- Chicken Broth (41 Calories)

- Beef Broth (10 Calories)

- Tea (nothing added) (2.4 Calories)

- Coffee (nothing added) (1.8 Calories)

Note: This is a 24-hour fast. No food is to be consumed during this time. It is advised to only choose from the options above. Stay within your caloric intake. This meal plan is just an EXAMPLE of what your Mondays should look like.

BREAKFAST:

EGG WHITE AVOCADO AND TOMATO SCRAMBLE

- 4 EGG WHITES
- 1 MEDIUM RAW PLUM TOMATO
- ½ FRUIT AVOCADO
- 1 DASH OF SALT
- 1 DASH OF PEPPER
- 1 TSP SRIRACHA SAUCE

1. Turn on stove to medium heat and spray cooking spray in the pan. Whisk the egg whites with salt and pepper.
2. Chop tomato and avocado and set it aside.
3. Add tomatoes and cook for one minute.
4. Remove eggs from pan and add avocado, another dash of salt, pepper and sriracha on top.

LUNCH:

SMOKED SALMON AND CUCUMBER SALAD

- ¼ CUP CHOPPED SCALLIONS
- 1 TSP DILL
- ½ TBSP DRAINED CAPERS
- 2 TSP MAYONNAISE
- 1.3 OZ CUCUMBER
- 3 OZ CHINOOK SALMON
- ¼ TSP SALT
- ¼ TSP PEPPER

1. Combine the green onions, dill, capers, and mayonnaise mixture.
2. Chop cucumber into small pieces and add to the mixture.
3. Coarsely chop the salmon into chunks and add to mayonnaise mixture, while giving it a

good stir. Season to taste with salt and pepper.

CINNAMON APPLE BITES

- 1 MEDIUM APPLE
- ½ TSP CINNAMON

1. Cut up apples (without skin) into bite-sized chunks and add them into a container with a lid.
2. Sprinkle the cinnamon on top, close the lid, and gently shake.
3. Enjoy immediately.

Continued on next page…

DINNER:
MAPLE GLAZED CHICKEN

- ½ TBSP MAPLE SYRUP
- ½ TBSP HOISIN SAUCE
- ½ TSP DIJON MUSTARD
- 1 DASH OF PEPPER
- ½ TSP VEGETABLE OIL
- 2 OZ CHICKEN BREAST (BONELESS)

1. Preheat oven to 400 degrees, while combining the first 4 ingredients into a bowl; stir with a whisk.
2. Place the chicken in the broiler pan and cover with oil.
3. Brush it with maple mixture and bake for 10- 15 minutes, brushing with mixture after 5

min. and again after 10 min. Cook until juices run clear, chicken is no longer pink.

KALE CHIPS
- 2 CUP CHOPPED KALE
- ½ TBSP OLIVE OIL
- 1 DASH OF SALT

1. Preheat oven 350 degrees.
2. Remove center ribs and stems from kale (if present).
3. Tear kale leaves into 3 to 4-inch pieces.
4. Toss kale leaves in olive oil and salt. Spread on baking sheet that is coated with cooking
spray.
5. Bake for 12-15 minutes at 350 degrees until browned around the edge and crisp. Enjoy!

SNACK:
FRESH STRAWBERRY LIMEADE
- .6 OZ STRAWBERRIES
- .9 OZ FRUIT LIMES
- .3 OZ RAW AGAVE NECTAR
- ¼ CUP WATER
- 4 ¼ FL. OZ CLUB SODA

1. Add fresh strawberries, limes, agave, and water to a blender and blend until smooth.
2. Using a strainer to catch all the chunks, pour strawberry lime mixture.
3. Add club soda to strawberry limeade and finish off with ice.

ALMOND BUTTER AND CELERY
- 2 TBSP ALMOND BUTTER
- 2 STALKS CELERY

1. Spread almond butter on the celery.

BREAKFAST:

2 BANANA EGG PANCAKES
- 1 MEDIUM BANANA
- 2 LARGE EGGS

1. Mash the ripe banana.
2. Beat the eggs and stir in the banana.
3. Pour into lightly oiled frying pan. Flip when bubbles form.
4. Usually every 2 eggs/ 1 banana, makes 2 small pancakes.

LUNCH:

TUNA SALAD
- ½ CAN TUNA
- ½ FRUIT AVOCADO
- ½ TBSP LEMON JUICE
- .3 OZ CHOPPED ONION

1. Mix and mash all ingredients, then add salt, pepper, and garlic powder to your preference.

SLICED BELL PEPPER
- 1 MEDIUM RED BELL PEPPER

1. Wash the bell pepper, slice it in half, then remove seeds and stem.
2. Slice into strips and enjoy!
3. Optional: enjoy with a side of hummus/dip

DINNER:

CHICKEN STIR-FRY
- 1 DASH CAYENNE PEPPER
- 2 OZ CHICKEN BREAST
- 1 TSP CHICKEN BROTH
- ¼ CUP ASPARAGUS
- ¼ CUP CHOPPED BROCCOLI
- ¼ CUP GINGER
- ½ CUP SLICED MUSHROOMS
- ¼ CARROT
- .5 OZ EGG

1. Heat the chicken stock or broth in a nonstick wok over medium high heat.
2. Chop the vegetables.
3. Cut the chicken into strips or chunks and add to the wok (or any other protein choice)
4. Cook until almost done.
5. Add the vegetables, cayenne pepper, and ginger, cook until tender.
6. Separately, quickly scramble the egg and then add to the stir fry.
7. Serve hot and enjoy!

CARROTS
- 1 CUP BABY CARROTS

1. Enjoy by themselves or with a side of hummus.

Continued on next page…

SNACK:

BASIC MIXED GREEN SALAD
- 1 CUP SHREDDED LETTUCE
- 1 SERVING MIXED BABY GREENS
- 1/4 CUP SHREDDED RADICCHIO
- ½ CUP PARSLEY
- ¼ CUP ARUGULA

1. Mix all greens in a bowl, top it with a little of your favorite dressing.

SNACK:

ALMONDS
- 1 OZ. ALMONDS (23 KERNELS)

1. Enjoy!

BREAKFAST:

2 INGREDIENT PROTEIN PANCAKES	
• ½ CUP MASHED BANANA • 1 JUMBO EGG • 3 EGG WHITES (SEPARATED FROM YOLK)	1. Mash the banana and crack the eggs into it, stir until well blended. 2. Heat a greased griddle on medium heat and pour about a 2.5-inch puddle of batter. 3. Carefully flip the pancake after about 25 seconds or when it browns. 4. Flip and finish browning other side. 5. Repeat with remaining batter and enjoy! (Recipe from bodybuilding.com)
BACON	
• 2 STRIPS BACON	1. Cook bacon in a skillet over medium high heat until brown and crisp, turning to brown evenly.

LUNCH:

CURRY TUNA SALAD	
• ½ CAN OF TUNA • 1 TBS OF MAYONNAISE • 1 TBS CHOPPED ONION • ¼ TSP SALT	1. Chop onions. 2. Drain tuna. 3. Add all ingredients together.
ALMONDS	
• 1 OZ. (23 WHOLE KERNELS)	1. Enjoy!

DINNER:

ZUCCHINI NOODLES	
• 1 LARGE ZUCCHINI • ½ SMALL ONION • 1 CLOVE GARLIC, MINCED • ½ TSP SALT • ½ TSP PEPPER	1. Peel the Zucchini and cut them into wide julienne strips or noodles with a mandolin or a spiralizer. 2. Add onion, garlic, salt, and pepper to a medium sauce pan, over medium heat. 3. Cook over medium heat for 1-2 minutes, until fragrant and slightly softened. 4. Toss with zucchini noodles and cook for 1-2 minutes until evenly heated through.

Continued on next page…

KALE CHIPS
- 2 CUPS CHOPPED KALE
- ½ TBSP OLIVE OIL
- PINCH OF SALT

1. Preheat oven to 350 degrees and remove center ribs and stems from kale if present. Tear kale leaves into 3-4-inch pieces.
2. Toss kale leaves into olive oil and salt, spread on baking sheet coated with cooking spray.
3. Bake 12-15 minutes until crisp and brown on edges.

SNACK:

COOL SUMMER CUCUMBER CHICKEN AND TOMATO TOSS
- 70 GRAMS LARGE CUCUMBER
- ½ LARGE TOMATO
- 2 SPRIGS OF FRESH CILANTRO
- 1 TBSP OF LEMON JUICE
- ¼ CAN CHICKEN
- 1 DASH OF PEPPER AND SALT

1. Place cucumber, tomatoes, and cilantro in a bowl.
2. Season with lemon juice, salt and pepper. Toss gently to coat evenly. Add canned chicken and toss again. Serve immediately or refrigerate until ready to serve.

CARROTS
- 1 CUP BABY CARROTS

1. Enjoy!

BREAKFAST:

ANTI-INFLAMMATORY TURMERIC GINGER TONIC • 2 TBSP WATER • 1/2 TSP GINGER • 1/2 TSP TURMERIC • 1/2 TSP CINNAMON	1. Bring water to boil. 2. Add spices and simmer for up to 10 minutes.
EASY HARD-BOILED EGGS • 3 LARGE EGGS	1. Place eggs in a pot and cover completely with water. 2. Cover and turn stove on high, bring to a boil, turn off heat and place pot on cool burner. Let the pot sit with cover on it for 15 minutes. 3. Meanwhile; Fill a large bowl halfway with cold water, transfer the eggs from the pot to the cold water. 4. Replace the water as needed to keep cold until the eggs are completely cooled. 5. Chill in refrigerator at least 2 hours before peeling.

LUNCH:

LIME CHICKEN SALAD • 1 CAN OF CHICKEN • 2 TSP LIME JUICE • 1 DASH OF SALT • 4 LARGE LETTUCE LEAFS	1. Combine the chicken, lime juice, and salt. 2. Arrange the lettuce leaves and serve the chicken salad on top.
BANANA • 1 MEDIUM SIZE BANANA	1. Enjoy!

Continued on next page…

DINNER:

SHRIMP WITH CAULIFLOWER AND BOK CHOY

- 1 CLOVE GARLIC MINCED
- 2 3/4 OZ SHRIMP
- ½ CUP CHOPPED CABBAGE (BOK CHOY)
- 1 DASH OF SALT
- 2 TSP OLIVE OIL
- 1 DASH OF PEPPER
- 1 RAW RED CHILLI PEPPER
- ¼ CUP FRESH CILANTRO

1. Sauté garlic and shrimp in oil for 3-4 minutes. Add in cabbage (bok choy).
2. Season with salt, pepper and chili peppers.
3. Stir until cooked bok choy is tender. Do not overcook. Top with cilantro.

SNACK:

ALMOND BUTTER AND CELERY

- 2 TBSP ALMOND BUTTER
- 2 LARGE STALKS OF CELERY

1. Spread almond butter on celery and enjoy!

BREAKFAST:

SOUTHWEST SALSA EGGS

- 1 SPRITZ OF PAM COOKING SPRAY
- 2 LARGE EGGS
- 1 TBSP SALSA

1. Use some vegetable spray to coat the pan. Allow it to warm up on medium heat.
2. Put the eggs in the pan and scramble.
3. Lower the heat.
4. Add salsa.
5. Stir until firm and enjoy!

FRUIT SALAD

- 1 CUP OF HALVED STRAWBERRIES
- 1 CUP BLUEBERRIES

1. Mix together and enjoy!

LUNCH:

TURKEY KIELBASA HASH

- 5 OZ HASHBROWN
- 1 SERVING KIELBASA SAUSAGE (2OZ)
- 1 TBSP OLIVE OIL
- .6 OZ RED BELL PEPPER
- .3 OZ GREEN BELL PEPPER
- .5 OZ ONION
- 1 DASH OF SALT
- 1 DASH OF PEPPER

1. Cook hash browns according to package directions.
2. In a separate skillet, brown the sliced kielbasa for around 5 minutes in 1 tbsp of olive oil over medium-high heat.
3. Remove kielbasa from pan and set aside. Add the peppers and onions to the skillet and season with a pinch of salt and pepper. Cook for 5 minutes, or until softened, stirring occasionally.
4. Add hash browns and kielbasa to skillet with the onions and peppers and mix everything together. Serve hot and enjoy!

FRIED BROCCOLI

- ¼ PACKAGE OF BROCCOLI
- ¼ TBSP OLIVE OIL
- 1 DASH CRUSHED RED PEPPER FLAKES
- ¼ TSP SALT

1. Rinse and pat dry broccoli.
2. Heat the olive oil in a large skillet over medium heat, add red peppers and heat for 1 minute.
3. Cook and stir broccoli in the skillet until it begins to get crispy, 5-7 minutes. Season with salt to serve.

Continued on next page…

DINNER:
ZUCCHINI NOODLES

- 1 LARGE ZUCCHINI
- ½ SMALL ONION
- 1 CLOVE GARLIC MINCED
- ½ TSP SALT
- ½ TSP PEPPER

1. Peel the zucchini and cut them into wide julienne strips or noodles with a mandolin or a spiralizer.
2. Add onion, garlic, salt, and pepper, to a sauce pan, over medium heat.
3. Cook over medium heat for 1-2 minutes, until fragrant and slightly softened.
4. Toss with zucchini noodles and cook for 12 minutes, until evenly heated.

SNACK:
TURKEY AND AVOCADO WRAP

- ¼ FRUIT AVOCADO
- 2 OZ DELI CUT TURKEY

1. Core and cut avocado.
2. Wrap avocado in turkey.

ote: Above is one full day "substitute" meal plan that can be used to terchange any day in Restore week (Tuesday through Friday). Choose is substitute meal plan if you want and substitute it in for any day you 10ose.

BREAKFAST:

BANANA AND KALE SMOOTHIE
- 1 CUP COCONUT WATER (LIQUID FROM COCONUT)
- ½ CUP BANANA
- 1 CUP KALE
- ½ OZ CHIA SEEDS
- ¾ CUP BLUEBERRIES

1. Combine all ingredients in a blender and pulse until smooth.

LUNCH:

DEVILED EGG SALAD
- 2.5 GRAMS VINEGAR
- 2 EXTRA LARGE EGGS
- 1 DASH SALT
- 1 DASH PEPPER OR HOT SAUCE
- .3 OZ CHOPPED CELERY
- ½ TBSP DIJON MUSTARD
- 1 DASH OF PEPPER
- 1/2 TSP PAPRIKA
- 1 TBSP LIGHT MAYONNAISE
- .4 OZ CHOPPED RED BELL PEPPER
- 1 TSP CHOPPED SCALLIONS

1. Hard boil and then peel eggs. Chop green onion, celery, and red bell pepper coarsely.
2. Chop the eggs coarsely and put them into a large bowl. Add green onion, celery, red bell pepper.
3. In a small bowl mix the mayonnaise, mustard, vinegar, and hot sauce. Gently stir the mayo dressing into the bowl with the eggs and vegetables.
4. Add paprika and salt and black pepper to taste. Best served chilled.

ROASTED ASPARAGUS
- 6 ASPARAGUS SPEARS
- 1 DASH SALT
- 1 TSP OLIVE OIL

1. Preheat oven to 425 degrees and cut off the bottom part of asparagus spears and discard.
2. With a vegetable peeler, peel off the skin on the bottom 2-3 inches of the spears.
3. Place asparagus on foil lined baking sheet and drizzle with olive oil. Sprinkle with salt.
4. Roll the asparagus around until they are evenly coated.
5. Roast for 10-15 minutes, depending on the thickness of the stalk and how tender you prefer. Should be tender when pierced with a knife.

Continued on next page…

DINNER:

FILET MIGNON WITH RICH BALSAMIC GLAZE

- 2 BEEF TENDERLOIN 4 OZ. EACH
- ½ TSP PEPPER
- 1 TSP SALT
- 4 TBSP BALSAMIC VINEGAR
- 1 FL OZ RED WINE

1. Sprinkle freshly ground pepper and salt over both sides of steaks. Heat a nonstick skillet over medium-high heat.
2. Place steaks in hot pan, and cook for 1 minute on each side, or until browned. Reduce heat to medium-low and add balsamic vinegar and red wine. Cover and cook for 4 minutes on each side, basting with sauce when flipping over.
3. Remove steaks to two warm plates, spoon 1 tbsp of glaze over each steak and serve immediately.

FRIED BROCCOLI

- 4 OZ BROCCOLI
- 1 TSP OLIVE OIL
- 1 DASH CRUSHED RED PEPPER FLAKES
- ¼ TSP SALT

1. Rinse and pat dry broccoli.
2. Heat olive oil in a large skillet over medium heat, add crushed red pepper flakes and heat 1 minute.
3. Cook and stir broccoli in a skillet until it begins to get crispy, 5-7 minutes. Season with salt and serve.

SNACK:

MANGO STRAWBERRY ARUGULA SALAD

- 3 CUPS ARUGULA
- ½ MANGO, SLICED
- ½ CUP SLICED STRAWBERRIES
- ½ FRUIT AVOCADO
- ¼ MEDIUM ONION

1. Place arugula in a bowl. Top with sliced mango, sliced strawberries, sliced avocado, and then sliced red onion.
2. Top with dressing of your choice.

<u>Note:</u> Above is one full day "substitute" meal plan that can be used to interchange any day in Restore week (Tuesday through Friday). Choose this substitute meal plan if you want and substitute it in for any day you choose.

FOOD ITEM	AVERAGE SERVING SIZE	CALORIES
PROTEIN		
HAMBURGER PATTY	3.5 OZ	235 CAL
TRI TIP	3.5 OZ	182 CAL
PORK CUTLET	3.5 OZ	231 CAL
CHICKEN	4 OZ	190 CAL
BEEF NEW YORK STRIP STEAK	4 OZ	220 CAL
BABY BACK RIBS	3 OZ	270 CAL
PORK SIRLOIN	3 OZ	168 CAL
BEEF RIBEYE STEAK	6 OZ	450 CAL
SALMON	3 OZ	200 CAL
HALIBUT	3 OZ	107 CAL
FRIED EGG	1 LARGE EGG	92 CAL
BOILED EGG	1 LARGE EGG	77 CAL
SCRAMBLED EGG	1 LARGE EGG	101 CAL
CARBOHYDRATES		
BANANA	1 MEDIUM BANANA	104 CAL
APPLE	1 MEDIUM APPLE	80 CAL
ORANGE	1 FRUIT	69 CAL
SPAGHETTI WITH MEAT SAUCE	10 OZ	286 CAL
CHICKEN ALFREDO PASTA	8.14 OZ	321 CAL
WHITE RICE	1 CUP	205 CAL
BROWN RICE	1 CUP	216 CAL
BLACK BEANS	½ CUP	90 CAL
REFRIED BEANS	½ CUP	125 CAL
PINTO BEANS	½ CUP	144 CAL
BROCCOLI	1 CUP	65 CAL
GREEN BEANS	1 CUP	25 CAL
CORN	4 OZ	153 CAL
WHOLE WHEAT BREAD	1 SLICE	69 CAL
WHITE BREAD	1 SLICE	120 CAL
SOURDOUGH BREAD	1 SLICE	120 CAL
RESTAURANTS		
IN N OUT BURGER WITH ONION	1 SERVING	390 CAL

MCDONALDS CHEESEBURGER	1 SERVING	300 CAL
TACO BELL CRUNCHY SUPREME TACO	1 SERVING	190 CAL
TACO BELL BEAN BURRITO	1 SERVING	370 CAL
EL POLLO LOCO AL CARBON CHICKEN TACOS	1 SERVING	160 CAL
JAMBA JUICE ACAI PRIMO FRUIT BOWL	1 SERVING	540 CAL
CARL'S JR SPICY CHICKEN SANDWICH	1 SERVING	460 CAL
SUBWAY HAM SANDWICH 6 INCH	1 SERVING	450 CAL
PANERA BREAD STRAWBERRY POPPYSEED CHICKEN SALAD	1 SERVING	350 CAL
RED LOBSTER STARTER SAMPLER	1 SERVING	620 CAL
OLIVE GARDEN CHICKEN ALFREDO FETTUCCINE	1 SERVING	500 CAL
RED ROBIN WINGS	1 SERVING	1,023 CAL
APPLEBEE'S TRIPLE BACON BURGER	1 SERVING	1,190 CAL

Note: Above is an example of some but not all food items allowed in Combo. Remember you can eat anything you want in Combo (Saturday and Sunday) as long as you stay within your targeted caloric intake.

RECIPE: COMBO   *SATURDAY- SUNDAY: 1,000 CALORIES*

SATURDAY BREAKFAST:
- ½ CUP OATMEAL (PLAIN)
  (150 CALORIES)
- 70 CAL WHEAT BREAD
  (70 CALORIES)
- 1 TSP BUTTER

  (34 CALORIES)

SATURDAY LUNCH:
- GRILLED CHEESE SANDWICH
  (257 CALORIES)
- 7 COOL RANCH CHIPS
  (88 CALORIES)

SATURDAY DINNER:
- 7 OZ STOUFFER LASAGNA
  WITH MEAT
  (277 CALORIES)
- 1 OZ CORN BREAD SLICE
  (67 CALORIES)

SATURDAY SNACK:
- 1 SUGAR FREE JELLO CUP
  (5 CALORIES)
- .5 OZ POPCORN
  (50 CALORIES)

TOTAL: 998 CALORIES

SUNDAY BREAKFAST:
- 1 BUTTERMILK PANCAKE
  (175 CALORIES)
- 2 TBSP LITE SYRUP
  (53 CALORIES)

SUNDAY LUNCH:
- IN N OUT
  BURGER (195
  CALORIES)
- 1.5 OZ FRIES
  (126
  CALORIES)

SUNDAY DINNER:
- 1 CHEESE PIZZA SLICE
  (272 CALORIES)

SUNDAY SNACK:
- 1 MEDIUM GLAZED DONUT
  (192 CALORIES)

TOTAL: 1,012 CALORIES

<u>Note:</u> In Combo you can eat ANY food, but stay in your caloric intake!

Macro Circuit Recipe

1,300 Calorie Meal Plan

These meal plans are for those people who have the extra time to cook meals with recipes.

MONDAY BREAKFAST: (EXAMPLE 1)	MONDAY BREAKFAST: (EXAMPLE 2)
HOT BROTH • 12 OZ BEEF BROTH, HEATED	ORANGE JUICE • 12 OZ ORANGE JUICE (NO PULP)
LUNCH: APPLE JUICE • 12 OZ APPLE JUICE	LUNCH: GRAPE JUICE • 12 OZ GRAPE JUICE
DINNER: CRANBERRY JUICE • 12 OZ CRANBERRY JUICE	DINNER: TOMATO JUICE • 12 OZ TOMATO JUICE
SNACK: WATER • 12 OZ WATER	SNACK: VEGETABLE JUICE • 12 OZ VEGETABLE JUICE

<u>Reminder:</u> These are 2 examples of what your Mondays will look like. DO NOT FOLLOW THIS PLAN.

Things You Can Have During Your Flush: (Calories for 8 fl ounces)

- Coconut Water (46 Calories)

- Water (0 Calories)

- Carrot Juice (94 Calories)

- Apple Juice (105 Calories)

- Orange Juice (115 Calories)

- Grape Juice (152 Calories)

- Vegetable Juice (50 Calories)

- Pomegranate Juice (140 Calories)

- Tomato Juice (41 Calories)

- Grapefruit Juice (102 Calories)

- Cranberry Juice (116 Calories)

- Chicken Broth (41 Calories)

- Beef Broth (10 Calories)

- Tea (nothing added) (2.4 Calories)

- Coffee (nothing added) (1.8 Calories)

Note: This is a 24-hour fast. No food is to be consumed during this time. It is advised to only choose from the options above. Stay within your caloric intake. This meal plan is just an EXAMPLE of what your Mondays should look like.

BREAKFAST:

SCRAMBLED EGGS WITH BACON & MUSHROOM
- 2 EXTRA LARGE EGGS
- 2 STRIPS BACON
- ¼ CUP DICED MUSHROOMS

1. Cook the bacon over low heat, then remove from the pan, pat dry with paper towel, and put aside.
2. Rinse the mushrooms and pat them dry. Add mushrooms to a pan and cook over medium-low until soft.
3. Crack the eggs into a bowl and beat with a fork until thoroughly combined. Add the eggs to the pan of mushrooms and crumble the baked bacon into the pan as well.
4. Cook over medium-high until it begins to set, mixing the eggs with a spatula to ensure even cooking.

APPLE

- 1 APPLE

1. Enjoy!

LUNCH:

QUICK BUFFALO CHICKEN SALAD

- 2 TBSP PEPPER OR HOT SAUCE
- ½ CUP CANNED CHICKEN
- 1 CUP SPINACH
- 1 MEDIUM TOMATO (GREEN)

1. Mix hot sauce with chicken. Put on top of spinach and add tomatoes to the top.
2. Toss together and enjoy.

CARROTS
- 1 CUP BABY CARROTS

1. Enjoy!

DINNER:

HONEY GARLIC SALMON
- 4 OZ COHO SALMON
- 1 DASH OF SALT
- 1 DASH OF PEPPER
- 1 DASH OF CAYENNE PEPPER
- 2 TSP HONEY
- 1 TSP WATER

- ½ TSP LEMON JUICE
- 1 TSP OLIVE OIL
- 1 CLOVE, MINCED GARLIC
- 0.6 OZ LEMON JUICE

1. Season the salmon with salt, black pepper, and cayenne pepper and set aside.
2. Combine the honey, water, lemon juice, and a dash of salt together in a bowl and mix well.
3. Heat up a skillet and add the olive oil. Pan-fry the salmon until it is almost cooked. Add minced garlic into the pan and brown them.
4. Add the honey mixture and lemon wedges (optional) into the skillet and reduce the sauce until it's sticky.

Continued on next page…

GARLIC KALE

- ½ CUP, CHOPPED KALE
- ½ TBSP OLIVE OIL
- 1 CLOVE, MINCED GARLIC

1. Tear the kale leaves into bite sized pieces from the stems and discard them.
2. Heat the olive oil in a large pot over medium heat. Cook and stir the garlic in the hot oil until softened. (about 2 minutes)
3. Add the kale and continue cooking and stirring until the kale is bright green and wilted, about 5 minutes.

SNACK:

BASIC MIXED GREENS SALAD

- 1 CUP SHREDDED LETTUCE
- 1 CUP MIXED BABY GREENS
- 1/4 CUP SHREDDED RADICCHIO
- ½ CUP PARSLEY
- ¼ CUP ARUGULA

1. Mix all greens in a bowl, top it with a little of your favorite dressing.

SNACK:

ALMOND BUTTER AND CELERY

- 2 TBSP ALMOND BUTTER
- 2 STALKS CELERY

1. Spread almond butter on celery.

BREAKFAST:

PUMPKIN COCONUT PALEO SMOOTHIE	
<ul><li>½ CUP PUMPKIN</li><li>½ CUP COCONUT MILK</li><li>½ MEDIUM BANANA</li><li>1 DASH OF CINNAMON</li></ul>	1. Place all ingredients in the blender with 2- 3 ice cubes and blend until smooth. 2. (You do not need to use ice cubes if using a frozen banana.)

LUNCH:

CUCUMBER TOMATO SALAD WITH TUNA	
<ul><li>2 MEDIUM WHOLE TOMATOES</li><li>1 CUP SHREDDED LETTUCE</li><li>1 CUCUMBER</li><li>1 CAN OF LIGHT TUNA IN WATER</li></ul>	1. Chop vegetables and lettuce. 2. Toss together with the tuna.

DINNER:

MAPLE-GLAZED CHICKEN WITH APPLE BRUSSELS SPROUTS SLAW	
<ul><li>4 OZ CHICKEN BREAST</li><li>1 DASH OF SALT</li><li>1 DASH OF PEPPER</li><li>½ TBSP OLIVE OIL</li><li>2 TSP RED WINE VINEGAR</li><li>½ TBSP MAPLE SYRUP</li><li>2 OZ BRUSSELs SPROUTS</li><li>¼ MEDIUM APPLE</li><li>1 TBSP CURRANTS</li></ul>	1. Heat a large skillet over medium-high heat. Sprinkle chicken with salt and pepper. 2. Add oil to pan and cook the chicken for 4-7 minutes or until it is no longer pink. 3. Remove from pan and keep warm. Add vinegar and maple syrup to pan and bring to a boil. Cook for 1 minute or until it is reduced to 3 tablespoons. Return chicken to pan and turn to coat with glaze. 4. Cut Brussels sprouts in half lengthwise and thinly slice crosswise. Place remaining oil mixture in a large bowl and stir well. 5. Add Brussels sprouts, currants, and apple into bowl and toss to combine.

ZUCCHINI SPEARS	
<ul><li>1 DASH OF SALT</li><li>9 OZ ZUCCHINI</li></ul>	1. Cut zucchini lengthwise and then cut it into ¼ inch wedges. 2. Cook zucchini in boiling salt water until crisp-tender. (about 1 minute) 3. Drain and sprinkle with salt.

SNACK:

NUTRA-GREEN SALAD WITH BLACK FIG DRESSING	
<ul><li>1 ½ TBSP RED WINE VINEGAR</li><li>1 TBSP WATER</li><li>1 TSP DIJON MUSTARD</li><li>1 TSP ALMOND BUTTER</li><li>1 TSP KETCHUP</li><li>3 OZ MIXED BABY GREENS</li><li>¼ CUP ALFALFA SPROUTS</li><li>2 TBSP CHOPPED PECANS</li></ul>	1. Whisk together all ingredients except baby greens, sprouts and pecans, until smooth. 2. Toss salad with dressing and serve topped with chopped pecans.

BANANA	
<ul><li>1 BANANA</li></ul>	1. Peel and enjoy!

BREAKFAST:

BASIC SCRAMBLED EGGS
- 3 LARGE EGGS
- ½ TBSP OLIVE OIL
- ½ TBSP CHOPPED CHIVES
- ½ TBSP GROUND TARRAGON
- 1 DASH OF SALT
- 1 DASH OF PEPPER

1. Whisk eggs, salt, and pepper into medium bowl until eggs are broken up. Place 2 tablespoons of the eggs in a small bowl and set it aside.
2. Heat a 10-inch nonstick frying pan over medium-low until hot. (about 2 minutes)
3. Pour in the large portion of the eggs and sprinkle with chives and or tarragon and let sit undisturbed until eggs just start to set around the edges. (about 2 minutes)
4. Using the rubber spatula, push the eggs from the edges into the center. Let sit again for about 30 seconds, then repeat step.
5. Add remaining raw eggs and stir until eggs no longer look wet. Remove from heat and season.

BLUEBERRIES
- 1 CUP BLUEBERRIES

1. Enjoy!

LUNCH:

CHICKEN CELERY STICKS
- 1 CAN CHICKEN (5 OZ)
- 2 TBSP LIGHT MAYONNAISE
- ½ TSP GARLIC POWDER
- 1 DASH OF SALT
- 2 TSP PEPPER OR HOT SAUCE
- 3 STALKS, LARGE CELERY

1. Combine chicken, mayo, garlic powder, salt, and hot sauce in a small bowl and mix until well combined.
2. Cut celery stalks in half and stuff each one with the chicken mixture.

CARROTS
- 1 CUP BABY CARROTS

1. Enjoy!

DINNER:

ZUCCHINI NOODLES WITH MEAT AND MUSHROOM TOMATO SAUCE
- ½ LARGE ZUCCHINI
- ½ TBSP OLIVE OIL
- 3 TBSP CHOPPED ONIONS
- 1/3 CUP GARLIC
- 2 TBSP DICED MUSHROOM
- 3 OZ GROUND TURKEY
- 2 OZ PLUM TOMATO
- 1 TSP TOMATO PASTE
- 1 DASH OF SALT
- 1 DASH OF PEPPER
- 3 TBSP BASIL LEAVES

1. Run large zucchini through a spiralizer to create noodles. (If you don't have one, you can carefully use a peeler). Set aside.
2. Heat a large saucepan to medium-high heat.
3. Add olive oil and chopped onions to pan. Sauté until translucent. (about 2-3 minutes)
4. Add minced garlic cloves and sauté for 30 seconds and add sliced mushroom.
5. Cook until mushrooms are browned. (about 4-5 minutes)

Continued on next page…

6. Add ground turkey and sauté until cooked through. (about 6-10 minutes)
7. Add plum tomato and tomato paste, break up the tomatoes with a spoon in the pan. Season with salt and pepper.
8. Simmer sauce for 10 minutes.
9. In the meantime, heat a large skillet to medium-high heat.
10. Immediately add the zucchini noodles and flash sauté them for 2-3 minutes, stirring the whole time.
11. Remove from the pan and let sit, drain any excess water.
12. Finish off the meat mushroom sauce with freshly chopped basil.
13. Serve zucchini noodles with meat mushroom tomato sauce.

SNACK:

GINGER AND GREENS SMOOTHIE

- ½ CUP COCONUT WATER
- 1/3 CUP ICE CUBES
- ¼ CUP SLICED GINGER ROOT
- 1 CUP, CHOPPED KALE
- ¼ CUP FRESH CILANTRO
- ¼ FRUIT AVOCADO
- 2 KIWI FRUIT
- 1 TSP LIME JUICE

1. Combine all ingredients in a blender and pulse until smooth.

BREAKFAST:

2 INGREDIENT PROTEIN PANCAKES

- 2 LARGE EGGS
- 1 SPRAY OF PAM COOKING SPRAY
- 1 MEDIUM BANANA

1. Peel the banana and break it up into several big chunks in a bowl using a dinner fork to thoroughly mash the banana. Continue mashing until the banana has a pudding-like consistency and no large lumps remain. (a few small lumps are okay) Once the banana is mashed, set it aside.
2. Crack eggs into a separate bowl and whisk the eggs together until the yolks and whites are completely combined.
3. Pour the eggs on top of the mashed banana and mix together. The batter will be very loose.
4. Heat a greased (grease with cooking spray) griddle on medium heat and drop roughly 2 tablespoons of batter onto the hot griddle. It should sizzle immediately and it doesn't turn up the heat slightly. Delicately flip the pancake after about 25 seconds or when it browns.
5. Transfer the cooked pancakes to a serving plate and continue cooking the rest of the batter. (Makes 8 small pancakes)

LUNCH:

TUNA SALAD

- ½ CAN TUNA
- ½ FRUIT AVOCADO
- ½ TBSP LEMON JUICE
- 2 TBSP CHOPPED ONIONS
- 1 DASH OF SALT
- 1 DASH OF PEPPER
- 1 DASH OF GARLIC POWDER

1. Mix all ingredients together in a bowl and season with salt, pepper, and garlic powder.

BABY CARROTS

- 1 CUP BABY CARROTS

1. Enjoy!

Continued on next page…

DINNER:

FILET MIGNON WITH RICH BALSAMIC GLAZE

- 4 OZ BEEF TENDERLOIN
- ¼ TSP PEPPER
- ½ TSP SALT
- 1 FL OZ RED WINE
- 2 TBSP BALSAMIC VINEGAR

1. Sprinkle pepper over both sides of beef tenderloin and sprinkle with salt. Heat a nonstick skillet over medium-high heat.
2. Place steaks in hot pan, and cook for 1 minute on each side, or until browned. Reduce heat to medium-low and add balsamic vinegar and red wine. Cover and cook for 4 minutes on each side, basting with the sauce when you turn the meat over.
3. Remove the steaks to two warmed plates and pour 1 tbsp of glaze over each one. Serve immediately.

BACHELOR BRUSSELS SPROUTS

- 1 CUP BRUSSELS SPROUTS
- 1 DASH OF SALT
- 1 TBSP COCONUT OIL

1. Wash sprouts. Cut and discard the stems and then split them in half-length wise.
2. Heat coconut oil in frying pan on medium and add Brussels sprout halves and season while stirring to coat evenly.
3. Cook until slightly charred on edges. Allow them to cool and then serve.

SNACK:

EASY TOSSED SALAD

- 1 CUP SHREDDED LETTUCE
- 1 MEDIUM WHOLE TOMATO
- 1 LARGE CARROT
- 1 CUCUMBER
- 1 MEDIUM SCALLION
- 1 TBSP RANCH DRESSING

1. Chop lettuce, tomato, carrots, cucumber, and scallions. Toss it all together with a little dressing of your choice.

ALMONDS

- 1 OZ ALMONDS (23 KERNELS)

1. Enjoy!

BREAKFAST:

SIMPLE SPINACH SCRAMBLE

- 2 TSP OLIVE OIL
- 1 CUP SPINACH
- ¼ CUP CHOPPED ONIONS
- 2 RINGS OF BELL PEPPER
- 2 LARGE EGG
- 1 DASH OF SALT
- 1 DASH OF PEPPER

1. Clean the spinach off and throw it into a pan while it's still wet. Cook on medium heat and season with salt and pepper.
2. Once the spinach is wilted add the onion and peppers and cook until the onions are translucent and the pepper chunks are soft.
3. Add the eggs and scramble until cooked. Top with salt and pepper.

Excerpt From: Michael Matthews The Shredded Chef iBook http://itun.es/ca/V7n-F1

BACON

- 4 STRIPS BACON

1. Use a non-stick skillet and heat it on medium-high.
2. Add the bacon and cook, while occasionally flipping.
3. Cook to your preference.

LUNCH:

FRIED RIPE PLANTAINS

- 1 MEDIUM PLANTAINS
- 1 TBSP VEGETABLE OIL
- ½ DASH OF SALT

1. Peel the plantains and cut diagonally into ¼ inch thick slices.
2. Drizzle oil into a frying pan just enough to coat the bottom of the pan.
3. Place on medium heat.
4. When oil begins to simmer, add plantains. (work in batches)
5. Fry for 1 ½ minutes on one side then flip and cook for 1 minute on the other side.
6. Remove plantains from pan and rest on paper towels (to remove excess oil)
7. Continue frying in batches until all the plantains are fried.
8. Sprinkle lightly with salt to give a sweet and salty taste.

Continued on next page…

DINNER:

OVEN BAKED PALEO MEATBALLS

- 4 OZ GROUND BEEF
- ¼ MEDIUM ONIONS
- 2 TSP ROSEMARY
- 1 DASH OF SAGE
- 1 DASH OF SALT
- 1 DASH OF PEPPER
- 1/4 TSP CORIANDER SEED
- 1 TSP OLIVE OIL

1. Preheat oven to 400 degrees.
2. Line a sheet pan with foil or parchment paper and set it aside.
3. In a large skillet over medium heat, sauté the onions in oil until softened about 5 minutes.
4. Let cool.
5. In a large bowl combine the ground meat, onions and all the spices using your hands.
6. Form 2-inch balls and arrange them on the pan.
7. Bake for about 20 minutes or until cooked.

STEAMED CARROTS

- 1 LARGE CARROT
- 3 TBSP WATER
- 1 DASH OF SALT
- 1 DASH OF PEPPER

1. Bring water to a boil (about 1 to 2 inches, enough to create steam)
2. Cut up carrot into ½ inch pieces.
3. Place carrots in steaming basket and place the basket over the water. The carrots shouldn't be immersed in the water. You want the stem to cook them.
4. Steam carrots until done from 5-30 minutes depending on the carrot size.
5. Test the carrots to see if they are done by sticking a fork in them. It should slide in easily.

SNACK:

KIWI BERRY SMOOTHIE

- ½ CUP BLUEBERRIES
- ½ KIWI FRUIT
- ½ MEDIUM BANANA
- ½ CUP RASPBERRIES

1. Place all the ingredients in a blender and puree until smooth.

__Note:__ Above is one full day "substitute" meal plan that can be used to interchange any day in Restore week (Tuesday through Friday). Choose this substitute meal plan if you want and substitute it in for any day you choose.

BREAKFAST:

BAKED EGGS IN HAM	
• 2 SLICES OVAL HAM • 2 LARGE EGGS • 1 DASH OF SALT • 1 DASH OF PEPPER • 1 DASH OF PAPRIKA	1. Preheat oven to 375 degrees. Line a muffin tin with thick slices of ham. 2. Crack an egg into each muffin spot, and season with salt, pepper, and paprika. Bake for 20 minutes. 3. Slowly remove from muffin tin and enjoy! http://friskylemon.com/2012/02/01/bakedeggs-in-ham-cups

APPLE	
• 1 APPLE	1. Enjoy!

LUNCH:

ZUCCHINI NOODLES WITH MEAT AND MUSHROOM TOMATO SAUCE	
• ½ LARGE ZUCCHINI • ½ TBSP OLIVE OIL • 3 TBSP CHOPPED ONIONS • 1/3 CUP GARLIC • 2 TBSP DICED MUSHROOM • 3 OZ GROUND TURKEY • 1.8 OZ PLUM TOMATO • 1 TSP TOMATO PASTE • 1 DASH OF SALT AND PEPPER • 3 TBSP BASIL LEAVES	1. Run 3 large zucchinis through a spiralizer to create noodles. (If you don't have one, you can carefully use a peeler). Set aside. 2. Heat a large saucepan to medium-high heat. Add olive oil and chopped onions to pan. Sauté until translucent. (about 2-3 minutes) Add minced garlic cloves and sauté for 30 seconds and add sliced mushroom. 3. Cook until mushrooms are browned. (about 4-5 minutes) 4. Add ground turkey and sauté until cooked through. (about 6-10 minutes) 5. Add whole plum tomatoes and 2 tablespoons of tomato paste, break up the tomatoes with a spoon in the pot. Season with salt and pepper to taste. 6. Simmer sauce for 10 minutes. 7. In the meantime, heat a large skillet to medium high heat. 8. Immediately add the zucchini noodles and flash sauté them for 2-3 minutes, stirring the whole time. 9. Remove from pan and let sit, drain any excess water. 10. Finish off the meat mushroom sauce with freshly chopped basil. 11. Serve zucchini noodles with meat mushroom tomato sauce. Enjoy!

Continued on next page…

DINNER:

GRILLED ITALIAN SAUSAGE WITH PEPPERS, ONIONS, AND ARUGULA

- ½ TBSP OLIVE OIL
- 1 DASH OF SALT
- 2 TSP BALSAMIC VINEGAR
- ½ LARGE BELL PEPPER
- 1 CUP ARUGULA
- ¼ LARGE ONION
- 2 TSP HONEY
- 4 OZ ITALIAN SAUSAGE

1. Preheat grill. Mix together balsamic vinegar and honey in a small bowl and set it aside.
2. Coat the onion, pepper, and sausage with olive oil. Add a dash of salt. Coat the grill with a little olive oil. Put the onion wedges on the grill; cover. Let onions roast for 5 min. Turn the onions and move to a cooler part of the grill to finish.
3. If your grill has 2 levels. Place sausage on top part of the grill with the peppers below. If done this way the sausage juice and fat will drip on the peppers flavoring them.
4. If your grill doesn't have two levels, place the peppers on the hottest part of the grill and the sausage on the coolest.
5. Cover and grill for 15-20 minutes periodically checking.
6. Towards the end baste the sausage, peppers and onions with honey and balsamic mixture.
7. When done cooking remove from grill onto a pan.
8. Remove all or some charred skin on the peppers and cut them in long strips. Slice the root end of the onion off to help separate the pieces.
9. Cut the sausage into thirds. Mix everything and serve on top of a bed of baby arugula.

BACHELOR BRUSSELS SPROUTS

- 1 CUP BRUSSELS SPROUTS
- 1 DASH OF SALT AND PEPPER
- 1 TBSP COCONUT OIL

1. Wash sprouts and cut the stems off. Split the sprouts in half.
2. Heat coconut oil in frying pan on medium. Add Brussels sprout halves. Season them while stirring to coat evenly.
3. Cook until slightly charred on edges. Allow to cool; serve.

SNACK:

COOL SUMMER CUCUMBER CHICKEN AND TOMATO TOSS

- ¼ LARGE CUCUMBER
- ½ LARGE TOMATO
- 2 SPRIGS FRESH CILANTRO
- 1 TBSP LEMON JUICE
- 1 DASH OF SALT AND PEPPER
- ¼ CAN CHICKEN (5 OZ)

1. Place cucumber, tomatoes, and cilantro in a bowl. Season with lemon juice, salt and pepper. Toss gently to coat.
2. Add canned chicken and toss.
3. Serve immediately.

BABY CARROTS

- 1 CUP BABY CARROTS

1. Enjoy!

Note: Above is one full day "substitute" meal plan that can be used to interchange any day in Restore week (Tuesday through Friday). Choose this substitute meal plan if you want and substitute it in for any day you choose.

FOOD ITEM	AVERAGE SERVING SIZE	CALORIES
PROTEIN		
HAMBURGER PATTY	3.5 OZ	235 CAL
TRI TIP	3.5 OZ	182 CAL
PORK CUTLET	3.5 OZ	231 CAL
CHICKEN	4 OZ	190 CAL
BEEF NEW YORK STRIP STEAK	4 OZ	220 CAL
BABY BACK RIBS	3 OZ	270 CAL
PORK SIRLOIN	3 OZ	168 CAL
BEEF RIBEYE STEAK	6 OZ	450 CAL
SALMON	3 OZ	200 CAL
HALIBUT	3 OZ	107 CAL
FRIED EGG	1 LARGE EGG	92 CAL
BOILED EGG	1 LARGE EGG	77 CAL
SCRAMBLED EGG	1 LARGE EGG	101 CAL
CARBOHYDRATES		
BANANA	1 MEDIUM BANANA	104 CAL
APPLE	1 MEDIUM APPLE	80 CAL
ORANGE	1 FRUIT	69 CAL
SPAGHETTI WITH MEAT SAUCE	10 OZ	286 CAL
CHICKEN ALFREDO PASTA	8.14 OZ	321 CAL
WHITE RICE	1 CUP	205 CAL
BROWN RICE	1 CUP	216 CAL
BLACK BEANS	½ CUP	90 CAL
REFRIED BEANS	½ CUP	125 CAL
PINTO BEANS	½ CUP	144 CAL
BROCCOLI	1 CUP	65 CAL
GREEN BEANS	1 CUP	25 CAL
CORN	4 OZ	153 CAL
WHOLE WHEAT BREAD	1 SLICE	69 CAL
WHITE BREAD	1 SLICE	120 CAL
SOURDOUGH BREAD	1 SLICE	120 CAL
RESTAURANTS		
IN N OUT BURGER WITH ONION	1 SERVING	390 CAL

MCDONALDS CHEESEBURGER	1 SERVING	300 CAL
TACO BELL CRUNCHY SUPREME TACO	1 SERVING	190 CAL
TACO BELL BEAN BURRITO	1 SERVING	370 CAL
EL POLLO LOCO AL CARBON CHICKEN TACOS	1 SERVING	160 CAL
JAMBA JUICE ACAI PRIMO FRUIT BOWL	1 SERVING	540 CAL
CARL'S JR SPICY CHICKEN SANDWICH	1 SERVING	460 CAL
SUBWAY HAM SANDWICH 6 INCH	1 SERVING	450 CAL
PANERA BREAD STRAWBERRY POPPYSEED CHICKEN SALAD	1 SERVING	350 CAL
RED LOBSTER STARTER SAMPLER	1 SERVING	620 CAL
OLIVE GARDEN CHICKEN ALFREDO FETTUCCINE	1 SERVING	500 CAL
RED ROBIN WINGS	1 SERVING	1,023 CAL
APPLEBEE'S TRIPLE BACON BURGER	1 SERVING	1,190 CAL

Note: Above is an example of some but not all food items allowed in Combo. Remember you can eat anything you want in Combo (Saturday and Sunday) as long as you stay within your targeted caloric intake.

RECIPE: COMBO   *SATURDAY- SUNDAY: 1,300 CALORIES*

SATURDAY BREAKFAST:

- 2 CUPS HONEY NUT CHEERIOS CEREAL (293 CALORIES)
- 1 CUP MILK (108 CALORIES)

SATURDAY LUNCH:

- SUBWAY SANDWICH (450 CALORIES)

SATURDAY DINNER:

- 1 CUP HORMEL CHILI (260 CALORIES)
- 2 OZ CORNBREAD (198 CALORIES)

TOTAL: 1,310 CALORIES

SUNDAY BREAKFAST:

- 1 CUP GREEK GODS YOGURT (290 CALORIES)
- .5 OZ OATS GRANOLA (95 CALORIES)

SUNDAY LUNCH:

- 4 OZ CORN TORTILLA CHIPS (241 CALORIES)
- 10 OZ SALSA (71 CALORIES)

SUNDAY DINNER:

- 2 CUPS SPAGHETTI (347 CALORIES)
- 2 OZ FRENCH BREAD (188 CALORIES)

SUNDAY SNACK:

- 1 FAT FREE CHOCOLATE PUDDING CUP (100 CALORIES)

TOTAL: 1,333 CALORIES

<u>Note</u>: In Combo you can eat ANY food, but stay in your caloric intake!

Macro Circuit Recipe

1,500 Calorie Meal Plan

These meal plans are for those people who have the extra time to cook meals with recipes.

MONDAY BREAKFAST: (EXAMPLE 1)	MONDAY BREAKFAST: (EXAMPLE 2)
HOT BROTH • 12 OZ BEEF BROTH, HEATED	ORANGE JUICE • 12 OZ ORANGE JUICE (NO PULP)
LUNCH:	LUNCH:
APPLE JUICE • 12 OZ APPLE JUICE	GRAPE JUICE • 12 OZ GRAPE JUICE
DINNER:	DINNER:
CRANBERRY JUICE • 12 OZ CRANBERRY JUICE	TOMATO JUICE • 12 OZ TOMATO JUICE
SNACK:	SNACK:
WATER • 12 OZ WATER	VEGETABLE JUICE • 12 OZ VEGETABLE JUICE

<u>Reminder:</u> These are 2 examples of what your Mondays will look like. DO NOT FOLLOW THIS PLAN.

Things You Can Have During Your Flush: (Calories for 8 fl ounces)

- Coconut Water (46 Calories)
- Water (0 Calories)
- Carrot Juice (94 Calories)
- Apple Juice (105 Calories)
- Orange Juice (115 Calories)
- Grape Juice (152 Calories)
- Vegetable Juice (50 Calories)
- Pomegranate Juice (140 Calories)
- Tomato Juice (41 Calories)
- Grapefruit Juice (102 Calories)
- Cranberry Juice (116 Calories)
- Chicken Broth (41 Calories)
- Beef Broth (10 Calories)
- Tea (nothing added) (2.4 Calories)
- Coffee (nothing added) (1.8 Calories)

Note: This is a 24-hour fast. No food is to be consumed during this time. It is advised to only choose from the options above. Stay within your caloric intake. This meal plan is just an EXAMPLE of what your Mondays should look like.

BREAKFAST:

CARAMELIZED ONION FRITTATA
- 1 ½ EXTRA LARGE EGG
- 2 OZ ITALIAN SAUSAGE
- 1 DASH SALT AND PEPPER
- ¼ TBSP COCONUT OIL
- ½ MEDIUM ONION

1. Preheat oven to 350 degrees. Whisk eggs and thinly slice the onions. Cook Italian sausage in a large skillet over medium heat until cooked through.
2. Use a wooden spoon to break up the sausage while it cooks.
3. Grease a glass baking dish with the coconut oil. Place your Italian sausage in the dish.
4. While pan is still hot and over medium heat, add your sliced onions to the Italian sausage grease.
5. Cooking for about 8-10 minutes, continuously stirring onions to prevent burning.
6. While the onions are caramelizing, mix in your eggs with the Italian sausage in your baking dish.
7. Once the onions are caramelized, place the onions on top throughout the baking dish, covering all the eggs and Italian sausage.
8. Bake for 10-13 minutes or until your eggs are completely cooked through in the middle.

LUNCH:

CURRY TUNA SALAD
- ½ CAN TUNA
- 1 TBSP MAYONNAISE
- 1 TBSP CHOPPED ONIONS
- ¼ TSP SALT
- ¼ TSP CURRY POWDER

1. Chop onions. Drain Tuna. Add all ingredients together.

BANANA
- 1 MEDIUM SIZE BANANA

1. Enjoy!

DINNER:

QUICK AND SIMPLE STIR-FRIED KALE AND BACON
- 10 OZ KALE
- 6 STRIPS COOKED BACON
- 1 DASH SALT AND PEPPER
- 1 JUICE OF A LEMON WITHOUT SEEDS

1. Wash and chop the kale leaves, and prep remaining ingredients.
2. Sauté the bacon bits in a large cast iron skillet over medium heat. Once they are crisp add in the kale leaves, with a dash of salt and pepper.

Continued on next page…

3. Stir the kale and bacon for a couple minutes and then splash on some lemon juice.

SNACK:

SPICY CHICKEN CELERY STICKS

- 1 CAN CHICKEN (5 OZ)
- 2 TBSP LIGHT MAYONNAISE
- ½ TSP GARLIC POWDER
- ¼ TSP SALT
- 3 STALKS CELERY
- 2 TBSP HOT SAUCE

1. In a bowl, combine chicken, mayo, garlic powder, salt, and hot sauce together.
2. Cut celery stalks in half, stuff with chicken mixture.

SNACK:

CARROTS

- 1 CUP BABY CARROTS

1. Enjoy!

BREAKFAST:

PROTEIN SOUTHWEST SCRAMBLE
- 4 LARGE EGG WHITES
- 1.5 OZ SAUSAGE LINK
- 2 TSP OLIVE OIL
- 1 MEDIUM ONION
- ½ CUP CHOPPED RED BELL PEPPER
- 1 CUP SPINACH
- 1 MEDIUM WHOLE TOMATO
- 1 DASH OF SALT
- 1 DASH OF PEPPER

1. Dice the tomato, chop the red bell pepper, onion, and turkey sausage. In a large pan, drizzle onions and peppers with olive oil; sauté. When the onions are clear and peppers are tender, season with salt and pepper.
2. Add chopped turkey sausage, and sauté until sausage is golden brown. Lower heat, add egg whites, and scramble.
3. When eggs are almost done, add in tomato and spinach, mix around and then serve warm. (Recipe from bodybuilding.com)

BLUEBERRY WATERMELON SMOOTHIE
- 1 CUP DICED WATERMELON
- ½ CUP BLUEBERRIES
- 1 TSP LIME JUICE

1. Combine all ingredients in a blender and pulse until smooth. Add ice if desired.

LUNCH:

BALSAMIC RED WINE GLAZED FILET MIGNON
- 4 OZ BEEF TENDERLOIN
- ¼ TSP PEPPER
- ½ TSP SALT
- 2 TBSP BALSAMIC VINEGAR
- 1 OZ RED WINE

1. Sprinkle freshly ground black pepper over both sides of each steak, and sprinkle with salt to taste.
2. Heat a nonstick skillet over medium high heat. Place steaks in hot pan, and cook for 1 minute on each side, or until browned. Reduce heat to medium-low and add Balsamic vinegar and red wine. Cover, and cook for 4 minutes on each side, basting with sauce when flipping the meat over.
3. Remove steaks to two warmed plates, spoon one tablespoon of glaze over each, and serve immediately.

STEAMED BROCCOLI
- 6 OZ BROCCOLI
- 10 TBSP OLIVE OIL
- DROP OF LEMON JUICE

1. Trim broccoli into large florets and place it in a steaming basket over boiling water, cover and steam for 3 minutes.
2. Remove lid for a moment, then cook partially covered, until stems are tender-firm. (another 8-10 minutes)
3. Remove to platter, season with salt and pepper, olive oil, and lemon juice.

Continued on next page…

DINNER:

ZUCCHINI NOODLES WITH MEAT AND MUSHROOM TOMATO SAUCE

1. Run the zucchini through a spiralizer to create noodles. Heat a large saucepan to medium-

- ½ LARGE ZUCCHINI
- ½ TBSP OLIVE OIL
- 3 TBSP CHOPPED ONION
- 1/3 CUP CHOPPED GARLIC
- 2 TBSP DICED MUSHROOMS
- 3 OZ GROUND TURKEY
- 1.8 OZ OF A TOMATO
- 1 TSP TOMATO PASTE
- 1 DASH SALT
- 1 DASH PEPPER
- 3 TBSP FRESH BASIL LEAVES

1. high heat; add olive oil to pan, then the chopped onions. Sauté until translucent, about 2-3 minutes.
2. Add garlic and sauté for about 30 seconds, then add sliced mushrooms. Cook until mushrooms are brown, about 4-5 minutes.
3. Next add ground turkey and sauté until cooked through, about 6-10 minutes.
4. Add tomatoes and tomato paste, break up the tomatoes with a spoon in pot and add salt and pepper to taste.
5. Simmer sauce for 10 minutes. In the meantime, heat a large skillet to medium-high heat and immediately add zucchini noodles and flash sauté them for about 2-3 minutes, stirring the whole time. Remove from pan and let sit, drain any remaining water.
6. Finish off the meat mushroom sauce with some fresh basil.
7. Serve zucchini noodles with the meat mushroom sauce.

SNACK:

GRILLED POLENTA CHIPS
- 2 OZ OF YELLOW POLENTA
- 3.4 GRAMS OLIVE OIL
- ½ TBSP NUTRITIONAL YEAST
- 1 DASH OF PEPPER
- 1 DASH OF SALT

1. Heat a grill pan to medium-high heat and lightly rub your grill with olive oil.
2. Cut tube of polenta into ¼ inch to ½ inch slices. Brush both sides of the polenta cakes with the olive oil.
3. Sprinkle both sides with nutritional yeast, salt and pepper.
4. Lay the polenta rounds in one layer on the grill, and grill for 5 minutes on each side or until both sides are golden brown and crunchy with grill marks.
5. Remove the cakes from the grill and place on a large plate to cool. Serve warm or at room temperature.

TUNA SALAD AND SLICED RED BELL PEPPER
- ½ CAN OF TUNA
- ½ FRUIT AVOCADO
- ½ TBSP LEMON JUICE
- ¼ CUP CHOPPED ONION
- 1 MEDIUM RED BELL PEPPER

1. Mix and mash all ingredients, then add salt and pepper, and garlic powder to your preference.

BREAKFAST:

ENGLISH MUFFIN EGG SANDWICH

- ¼ TBSP OLIVE OIL
- 1 ENGLISH MUFFIN
- 1 LARGE EGG
- 1.8 OZ AVOCADO
- 1 DASH GARLIC POWDER
- 1 DASH CAYENNE PEPPER

1. Place skillet over medium heat and add olive oil, heat for 5 minutes. Place muffin in a toaster oven on toast setting.
2. Crack egg into pan, cooking for 3 minutes and flipping to cook 1 minute on the opposite side. Season with salt and pepper if desired.
3. Remove muffin from the toaster and place egg on bottom slice. Add sliced avocado and season with garlic powder and cayenne. Add second slice of muffin.

LUNCH:

PALEO AVOCADO CHICKEN SALAD

- 1 AVOCADO WITHOUT SKIN
- 1 LEMON YIELDS LEMON JUICE
- ¼ MEDIUM ONION
- 2 OZ PREMIUM CHUNKY CHICKEN BREAST
- 1 DASH OF SALT AND PEPPER

1. Cut the avocado in half and scoop the middle of both avocado halves into a bowl, leaving a shell of avocado flesh about ¼ inch thick on each half.
2. Add lemon juice and onion to the avocado in the bowl and mash together. Add drained chicken, salt and pepper, and stir to combine. Taste and adjust if needed.
3. Fill avocado shells with chicken salad and serve.

DINNER:

6 MINUTE SALMON

- 6 OZ SOCKEYE SALMON (BONELESS)
- 1 DASH OF SALT
- ½ TSP GARLIC POWDER
- ½ LEMON WITHOUT SEEDS

1. Preheat a cast iron skillet to high heat and set your oven to the broiler setting.
2. Take the filet of salmon and pat dry with a paper towel. Salt the skin side of the salmon and add it to the pan, skin side down.
3. Set the timer for two minutes. While the skin side is searing, season the other side generously with the garlic powder. Once the salmon is seared.
4. Place the cast iron into the oven for 4 minutes under the broiler.
5. Once the 4 minutes are up, serve the salmon with lemon wedges.

LEMON STEAMED BROCCOLI

- ¾ LB. BROCCOLI
- ½ TSP SALT
- ½ TSP PEPPER
- ½ TBSP OLIVE OIL
- ¼ TSP LEMON JUICE

1. Trim the broccoli into large florets.
2. Place the broccoli in a steaming basket over boiling water; cover and steam for 3 minutes.
3. Remove the lid for a moment, then cook, partially covered, until the stems are tender-firm, another 8-10 minutes. Remove to a platter, season with salt and pepper, olive oil, and lemon juice.

Continued on next page…

SNACK:

NUTRA-GREEN SALAD WITH BLACK FIG DRESSING

- 2 TBSP RED WINE VINEGAR
- 1 TBSP WATER
- ¼ TBSP DIJON MUSTARD
- ¼ TSP MARJORAM
- ¼ TBSP ALMOND BUTTER
- ¼ TBSP KETCHUP
- 3 OZ MIXED BABY GREENS
- ¼ CUP ALFALFA SPROUTS
- .5 OZ CHOPPED PECANS

1. Whisk together all ingredients except greens and pecans until smooth. Toss salad with dressing and serve topped with chopped pecans.

ALMOND BUTTER AND CELERY

- 2 TBSP ALMOND BUTTER
- 2 STALKS CELERY

1. Spread almond butter on celery stalks.

BREAKFAST:

EGG, AVOCADO, AND BACON SCRAMBLE	
<ul><li>2 STRIPS BACON</li><li>2 LARGE EGGS</li><li>3 EGG WHITES</li><li>¼ FRUIT AVOCADO</li></ul>	1. Cook bacon in a sauté pan over medium-high heat to desired crispiness. Remove from pan, reserving some grease. Chop bacon and set aside. 2. Add eggs and egg whites to the pan and cook until they begin to look less wet. Add the bacon and scramble until cooked through. Slice avocado and serve on top scramble.

APPLE	
<ul><li>1 APPLE</li></ul>	1. Enjoy!

LUNCH:

KETO SPICY TUNA ROLL	
<ul><li>1 SHEET SEAWEED</li><li>1 CAN TUNA</li><li>2 TBSP LIGHT MAYONNAISE</li><li>2 TBSP FRESH CILANTRO</li><li>2 TSP SRIRACHA SAUCE</li><li>¼ CUP FRUIT AVOCADO</li></ul>	1. Mix tuna, mayo, and cilantro in a bowl. Place seaweed sheet on a sushi mat with the rough non-shiny side facing up. If you do not have a sushi mat, lay a sheet of plastic wrap laid out on the counter. 2. Spread tuna mixture on bottom half of sheet. 3. Line avocado slices alongside the tuna. 4. Using the mat (or plastic wrap) roll the sheet over the tuna until it is rolled into a cylinder. 5. Apply a little pressure until the roll holds together on its own, then release it from the rolling mat. 6. Take a very sharp knife and slice the roll in to about 6 pieces. 7. Dot the top of each rill with a bit of Sriracha sauce.

STRAWBERRY PEAR JUICE	
<ul><li>1 MEDIUM PEAR</li><li>¼ CUP RASPBERRIES</li><li>¼ CUP STRAWBERRIES</li></ul>	1. Core pear. Juice ingredients and mix together well just before serving. Enjoy!

Continued on next page…

DINNER:

PINEAPPLE SHRIMP SALAD
- 4 OZ SHRIMP
- ½ TBSP OLIVE OIL
- 1 SMALL ONION
- ½ CUP PINEAPPLE CHUNKS
- ½ SMALL RED BELL PEPPER
- ½ FRUIT AVOCADO

1. Cook the shrimp with olive oil, salt and pepper over medium heat until bright pink and cooked through.
2. Toss together with remaining ingredients.

SNACK:

QUICK BUFFALO CHICKEN SALAD
- 2 TBSP HOT SAUCE
- ½ CUP CANNED CHICKEN
- 1 CUP SPINACH
- 1 MEDIUM GREEN TOMATO

1. Mix hot sauce with chicken. Put on top of spinach, add tomatoes on top.

CELERY
- 2 STALKS CELERY

1. Enjoy!

BREAKFAST:

SPINACH AND MUSHROOM EGG	
• 2 ½ LARGE EGGS • ½ DASH OF SALT • ½ DASH OF PEPPER • 4 CUPS SPINACH • ½ TBSP OLIVE OIL • 1 ¼ CUP MUSHROOMS	1. Whisk eggs together, season and set aside. 2. Fill a deep-frying pan with spinach, add olive oil and cover with a lid. Simmer and stir every so often for 5-10 minutes or until almost done. 3. Add mushrooms and continue cooking and stirring, cover until the mushrooms are lightly golden. Pour in the eggs and fry until the eggs are cooked through. Serve immediately.

APPLE	
• 1 MEDIUM APPLE	1. Enjoy!

LUNCH:

GRILLED ITALIAN SAUSAGE WITH PEPPERS, ONIONS, AND ARUGULA	
• ½ TBSP OLIVE OIL • ¼ DASH OF SALT • ¾ TBSP BALSAMIC VINEGAR • ½ LARGE RED BELL PEPPER • 1 CUP ARUGULA • ¼ LARGE ONION • ¾ TBSP HONEY • 4 OZ OF ITALIAN SAUSAGE	1. Preheat grill. Mix balsamic vinegar and honey in small bowl and set aside. Coat onion, peppers, and sausages with olive oil. Add salt to peppers and onions. Coat the grill with olive oil. 2. Put the onion wedges on the grill and cover. Let onions roast for 5 min, or until charred. Turn onions and move to cooler part of grill. 3. Put the peppers on the hottest part of the grill and the sausages on the coolest. Cover and grill everything for 15-20 min., periodically checking/turning sausages and peppers. 4. Towards the end of cooking, baste the sausages, peppers, and onions with honey balsamic mix. 5. When sausages, peppers and onions are cooked through, remove from grill and place on a pan. Cut peppers into long strips, slice root ends off onions to separate pieces. Cut sausages into thirds. 6. Mix everything and serve on bed of arugula.

TOMATO SOUP	
• ½ CAN TOMATO SOUP • ½ CUP WATER	1. Mix together condensed tomato soup and equal parts water. Microwave for 3 minutes, and then eat.

Continued on next page…

DINNER:

OVEN BAKED PALEO MEATBALLS
- 4 OZ GROUND BEEF
- ¼ MEDIUM ONION
- 1 DASH ROSEMARY
- 1 DASH SAGE
- 1 DASH CORIANDER SEED
- 1 DASH SALT
- 1 DASH PEPPER
- 1 TBSP OLIVE OIL

1. Preheat oven to 400 degrees. Line a sheet pan with foil or parchment paper and set aside.
2. In a large skillet over medium heat, sauté the onion in oil until softened, about 5 minutes.
3. Let cool. In a large bowl, combine the ground meat, onions and all the spices using your hands. Form into 2" balls and arrange on sheet pan.
4. Bake for about 20 minutes or until cooked through.

CARROTS
- 1 CUP BABY CARROTS

1. Enjoy by themselves. Optional, enjoy with a side of hummus.

SNACK:

PALEO AVOCADO CHICKEN SALAD
- 1 FRUIT AVOCADO
- 1 LEMON YIELDS JUICE
- ¼ MEDIUM ONION
- 2 OZ PREMIUM CHUNKY CHICKEN BREAST

1. Cut avocado in half and scoop the middle of avocados into a bowl, leaving a shell of avocado flesh about ¼ inch thick.
2. Add lemon juice and onion to avocado in the bowl and mash together. Add drained chicken, salt, pepper, stir to combine.
3. Fill avocado shells with chicken salad and serve.

CELERY
- 2 STALKS CELERY

1. Wash thoroughly and enjoy!

Note: Above is one full day "substitute" meal plan that can be used to interchange any day in Restore week (Tuesday through Friday). Choose this substitute meal plan if you want and substitute it in for any day you choose.

BREAKFAST:

KALE AND EGG CUPS	
<ul><li>1 TSP OLIVE OIL</li><li>8 OZ KALE</li><li>2 EXTRA LARGE EGGS</li><li>1 DASH OF SALT AND PEPPER</li></ul>	1. Preheat oven to 375 degrees and grease a muffin tin with olive oil. Set aside. 2. In a large pot, bring approximately 4 cups of water to a boil. Add the kale leaves and cook for about 1 minute. Have a large bowl of ice water standing by. 3. When the kale leaves have turned bright green and soft, remove from boiling water and immerse the leaves in the cold water to stop the cooking process. 4. Remove the cooled leaves from the ice water and pat dry with a paper towel. Line each cup of the muffin tin with a large kale leaf (trim the edge if necessary) 5. Into each kale lined cup, crack one egg. Sprinkle each with salt and pepper and bake for 20 minutes or until the egg is set. 6. Remove each egg cup from the muffin tin and serve them warm.
BACON<ul><li>2 STRIPS BACON</li></ul>	1. Cook bacon in a skillet over medium-high heat until browned and crisp, turning to brown evenly. 2. Bacon can also be cooked in the oven at 350 degrees for about 20 minutes, or microwave for about 50-60 seconds per strip.

LUNCH:

TURKEY LETTUCE ROLLUPS	
<ul><li>4 OUTER LEAF LETTUCE</li><li>4 SLICES OF DELI TURKEY</li><li>2 DASHES OF PEPPER</li></ul>	1. Lay out a large slice of lettuce, top with turkey. Sprinkle pepper over top and roll up. Repeat with remaining lettuce, turkey, and pepper.

Continued on next page…

DINNER:

GRILLED ITALIAN SAUSAGE WITH PEPPERS, ONIONS, AND ARUGULA

- ½ TBSP OLIVE OIL
- 1 DASH OF SALT
- .4 OZ BALSAMIC VINEGAR
- ½ LARGE RED BELL PEPPER
- 1 CUP ARUGULA
- .5 OZ GRAMS HONEY
- ¼ LARGE ONION CHOPPED IN WEDGES
- 4 OZ OF ITALIAN SAUSAGE

1. Preheat the grill. Mix together the balsamic vinegar and honey in a small bowl and set aside.
2. Coat the onion, peppers, and sausages with 2 tbsp. of olive oil. Add a dash of salt to the peppers and onions. Coat the grill with a little olive oil. Put the onion wedges on the grill, cover grill and let roast for 5 minutes, or until they are a little charred. Turn the onions and move them to a cooler part of the grill to finish.
3. Place the peppers on the hottest part of the grill and the sausages on the coolest. Cover everything and grill for 15-20 minutes. Periodically check and flip sausages and peppers when needed.
4. Toward the end of cooking, baste the sausages, peppers, and onion with the honey and balsamic mixture.
5. Remove everything from grill and transfer to a flat baking sheet, cut sausages into thirds, peppers into slices, cut root end off of onions and separate. Mix everything well in bowl.
6. To serve, place arugula on plate and top with sausage, onion and peppers.

Note: Above is one full day "substitute" meal plan that can be used to interchange any day in Restore week (Tuesday through Friday). Choose this substitute meal plan if you want and substitute it in for any day you choose.

FOOD ITEM	AVERAGE SERVING SIZE	CALORIES
PROTEIN		
HAMBURGER PATTY	3.5 OZ	235 CAL
TRI TIP	3.5 OZ	182 CAL
PORK CUTLET	3.5 OZ	231 CAL
CHICKEN	4 OZ	190 CAL
BEEF NEW YORK STRIP STEAK	4 OZ	220 CAL
BABY BACK RIBS	3 OZ	270 CAL
PORK SIRLOIN	3 OZ	168 CAL
BEEF RIBEYE STEAK	6 OZ	450 CAL
SALMON	3 OZ	200 CAL
HALIBUT	3 OZ	107 CAL
FRIED EGG	1 LARGE EGG	92 CAL
BOILED EGG	1 LARGE EGG	77 CAL
SCRAMBLED EGG	1 LARGE EGG	101 CAL
CARBOHYDRATES		
BANANA	1 MEDIUM BANANA	104 CAL
APPLE	1 MEDIUM APPLE	80 CAL
ORANGE	1 FRUIT	69 CAL
SPAGHETTI WITH MEAT SAUCE	10 OZ	286 CAL
CHICKEN ALFREDO PASTA	8.14 OZ	321 CAL
WHITE RICE	1 CUP	205 CAL
BROWN RICE	1 CUP	216 CAL
BLACK BEANS	½ CUP	90 CAL
REFRIED BEANS	½ CUP	125 CAL
PINTO BEANS	½ CUP	144 CAL
BROCCOLI	1 CUP	65 CAL
GREEN BEANS	1 CUP	25 CAL
CORN	4 OZ	153 CAL
WHOLE WHEAT BREAD	1 SLICE	69 CAL
WHITE BREAD	1 SLICE	120 CAL
SOURDOUGH BREAD	1 SLICE	120 CAL
RESTAURANTS		
IN N OUT BURGER WITH ONION	1 SERVING	390 CAL

MCDONALDS CHEESEBURGER	1 SERVING	300 CAL
TACO BELL CRUNCHY SUPREME TACO	1 SERVING	190 CAL
TACO BELL BEAN BURRITO	1 SERVING	370 CAL
EL POLLO LOCO AL CARBON CHICKEN TACOS	1 SERVING	160 CAL
JAMBA JUICE ACAI PRIMO FRUIT BOWL	1 SERVING	540 CAL
CARL'S JR SPICY CHICKEN SANDWICH	1 SERVING	460 CAL
SUBWAY HAM SANDWICH 6 INCH	1 SERVING	450 CAL
PANERA BREAD STRAWBERRY POPPYSEED CHICKEN SALAD	1 SERVING	350 CAL
RED LOBSTER STARTER SAMPLER	1 SERVING	620 CAL
OLIVE GARDEN CHICKEN ALFREDO FETTUCCINE	1 SERVING	500 CAL
RED ROBIN WINGS	1 SERVING	1,023 CAL
APPLEBEE'S TRIPLE BACON BURGER	1 SERVING	1,190 CAL

Note: Above is an example of some but not all food items allowed in Combo. Remember you can eat anything you want in Combo (Saturday and Sunday) as long as you stay within your targeted caloric intake.

RECIPE: COMBO   *SATURDAY- SUNDAY: 1,500 CALORIES*

| SATURDAY BREAKFAST: | SUNDAY BREAKFAST: |

SATURDAY BREAKFAST:
- 1 BREAKFAST BURRITO
  (302 CALORIES)

SATURDAY LUNCH:
- 1 AMIGOS MEXICAN RESTAURANT
  BURRITO
  (500 CALORIES)

SATURDAY DINNER:
- 1 FAST FOOD ENCHILADA
  WITH CHEESE
  AND BEEF
  (323 CALORIES)
- ½ CUP REFRIED BEANS
  (115 CALORIES)

SATURDAY SNACK:
- STARBUCKS CARAMEL MACCHIATO
  (190 CALORIES)

TOTAL: 1,429 CALORIES

SUNDAY BREAKFAST:
- 2 BUTTERMILK PANCAKES (6" DIA)
  (350 CALORIES)
- 4 TBSP LITE SYRUP
  (105 CALORIES)

SUNDAY LUNCH:
- 2 CRUNCHY TACOS, TACO BELL
  (340 CALORIES)

SUNDAY DINNER:
- 6 OZ ORANGE CHICKEN
  (399 CALORIES)

SUNDAY SNACK:
- 1 PIECE OF CHEESECAKE
  (257 CALORIES)
- 7 OZ STRAWBERRIES
  (64 CALORIES)

TOTAL: 1,515 CALORIES

<u>Note:</u> In Combo you can eat ANY food, but stay in your caloric intake!

<u>Macro Circuit Recipe</u>

1,800 Calorie Meal Plan

These meal plans are for those people who have the extra time to cook meals with recipes.

MONDAY BREAKFAST: (EXAMPLE 1)	MONDAY BREAKFAST: (EXAMPLE 2)

HOT BROTH
  • 12 OZ BEEF BROTH, HEATED
	ORANGE JUICE
	  • 12 OZ ORANGE JUICE (NO PULP)

LUNCH:	LUNCH:

APPLE JUICE
  • 12 OZ APPLE JUICE
	GRAPE JUICE
	  • 12 OZ GRAPE FRUIT

DINNER:	DINNER:

CRANBERRY JUICE
  • 12 OZ CRANBERRY JUICE
	TOMATO JUICE
	  • 12 OZ TOMATO JUICE

SNACK:	SNACK:

WATER
  • 12 OZ WATER
	VEGETABLE JUICE
	  • 12 OZ VEGETABLE JUICE

<u>Reminder:</u> These are 2 examples of what your Mondays will look like. DO NOT FOLLOW THIS PLAN.

Things You Can Have During Your Flush: (Calories for 8 fl ounces)

- Coconut Water (46 Calories)
- Water (0 Calories)
- Carrot Juice (94 Calories)
- Apple Juice (105 Calories)
- Orange Juice (115 Calories)
- Grape Juice (152 Calories)
- Vegetable Juice (50 Calories)
- Pomegranate Juice (140 Calories)
- Tomato Juice (41 Calories)
- Grapefruit Juice (102 Calories)
- Cranberry Juice (116 Calories)
- Chicken Broth (41 Calories)
- Beef Broth (10 Calories)
- Tea (nothing added) (2.4 Calories)
- Coffee (nothing added) (1.8 Calories)

Note: This is a 24-hour fast. No food is to be consumed during this time. It is advised to only choose from the options above. Stay within your caloric intake. This meal plan is just an EXAMPLE of what your Mondays should look like.

BREAKFAST:

SCRAMBLED EGGS WITH VEGETABLES
- 3 LARGE EGGS
- 1 DASH OF PEPPER
- 1 DASH OF SALT
- 1 ½ WHOLE MUSHROOM
- ¾ MEDIUM ONION
- 1 ½ TBSP OLIVE OIL

1. Scramble eggs with salt and pepper and set aside. Heat the pan to medium-low heat and add olive oil.
2. Add all the veggies to the pan and sauté lightly until almost soft.
3. Add scrambled eggs to the pan and let them sit till they begin to set.
4. Using the spatula, push the eggs from the side towards the middle. Repeat until eggs are cooked.

LUNCH:

CHICKEN CELERY STICKS
- 1 CAN OF CANNED CHICKEN
- 2 TBSP LIGHT MAYONNAISE
- ½ TSP GARLIC POWDER
- 1 DASH OF SALT
- 1 TSP OF PEPPER OR HOT SAUCE

1. Combine the chicken, mayo, pepper, salt, and garlic powder in a small bowl and mix until well combined.
2. Cut the celery stalks in half and stuff them with the chicken mixture.
3. Serve.

BANANA
- 1 BANANA

1. Peel and enjoy!

DINNER:

SHRIMP AND MUSHROOM ZOODLES
- ½ MEDIUM ZUCCHINI
- 2 TBSP OLIVE OIL
- 5 LARGE MUSHROOMS
- 6 OZ OF SHRIMP
- 2 CLOVES OF GARLIC
- ¼ TSP ONION POWDER
- ¼ TSP PAPRIKA
- 1 DASH OF SALT

1. Use a spiralizer to cut the zucchini into noodles, or use a peeler to carefully cut the noodles.
2. Add oil to a hot skillet over medium heat and sauté mushrooms until tender. Add shrimp, garlic, and spices and cook until the shrimp are carefully cooked. (3-4 minutes)
3. Remove shrimp and mushroom from the skillet then add the zucchini noodles and cook for about 2 minutes.
4. Remove from skillet and put it on a plate.

CARROTS
- 1 CUP BABY CARROTS

1. Enjoy!

Continued on next page…

COCONUT MANGO TROPICAL GREEN SMOOTHIE

- ¼ TSP STEVIA SWEETENER
- ½ MEDIUM BANANA
- 2 CUPS SPINACH
- 2 CUPS CHOPPED KALE
- 2 TBSP LIME JUICE
- ½ CUP SLICED MANGOS
- 1 CUP COCONUT WATER
- 1 OZ PLANT VEGAN PROTEIN

1. Combine all ingredients in a blender.
2. Blend and serve.

BREAKFAST:

PROTEIN SOUTHWEST SCRAMBLE

- 4 LARGE EGG WHITES
- ½ SAUSAGE LINK
- 2 TSP OLIVE OIL
- 1 MEDIUM ONION
- ½ CUP CHOPPED RED BELL PEPPER
- 1 CUP SPINACH
- 1 MEDIUM WHOLE TOMATO
- 1 DASH OF SALT
- 1 DASH OF PEPPER

1. Dice the tomato, chop the red pepper, onion, and turkey sausage.
2. In a large pan, drizzle the onions and peppers with olive oil and sauté. When the onions are clear and peppers are tender, season with salt and pepper.
3. Add chopped turkey sausage, and sauté until sausage is golden brown. Lower heat, add egg whites, and scramble.
4. When eggs are almost done, add in tomato and spinach, mix around, and then serve. Source: bodybuilding.com

APPLE

- 1 APPLE

1. Enjoy!

LUNCH:

CHICKEN KABOBS

- ½ CHICKEN BREAST
- ¼ LARGE GREEN BELL PEPPER
- ¼ LARGE ONION
- ¼ LARGE RED BELL PEPPER
- ¼ CUP BARBECUE SAUCE

1. Preheat the grill for high heat and slice the chicken breast into cubes to skew. Cut the onions and peppers into wedges to skew.
2. Thread the chicken, green bell pepper, onion, and red bell pepper onto skewers.
3. Lightly oil the grill grate. Place the kabobs on the prepared grill, and brush with barbecue sauce.
4. Cook, turning and brushing with the barbecue sauce frequently, for 15 minutes, or until the chicken juice runs clear.

CAULIFLOWER AND TAHINI

- 1 CUP CHOPPED CAULIFLOWER
- 2 TBSP SESAME TAHINI

1. Chop the cauliflower lovingly to retain some of the florets.
2. Serve with tahini for dipping.

Continued on next page…

DINNER:

PINEAPPLE SHRIMP SALAD

- 4 OZ SHRIMP
- ½ TBSP OLIVE OIL
- 1 SMALL ONION
- ½ CUP, CHUNKS PINEAPPLE
- ½ SMALL RED BELL PEPPER
- ½ FRUIT AVOCADO
- 1 LIME YIELDS LIME JUICE
- 1 CUP SHREDDED LETTUCE

1. Cook the shrimp with olive oil, salt and pepper over medium heat until bright pink and cooked through.
2. Toss together with other ingredients.

BACHELOR BRUSSELS SPROUTS

- 1 CUP BRUSSELS SPROUTS
- 1 TBSP COCONUT OIL

1. Wash sprouts and cut the stems off. Split the sprouts in half.
2. Heat coconut oil in frying pan on medium. Add Brussels sprout halves and season them stirring to coat evenly.
3. Cook until slightly charred on edges. Allow to cool.

SNACK:

KETO SPICY TUNA ROLL

- 1 SHEET SEAWEED
- 1 CAN OF TUNA
- 2 TBSP LIGHT MAYONNAISE
- 2 TBSP FRESH CILANTRO
- 2 TSP SRIRACHA SAUCE
- ¼ CUP, CUBED AVOCADO

1. Mix tuna, mayonnaise and cilantro in a bowl.
2. Place Nori seaweed sheet on a piece of plastic wrap laid out on the counter with the rough non-shiny side facing up. Spread the tuna mixture on bottom half of the sheet. Line avocado slices alongside the tuna.
3. Using the plastic wrap roll the sheet over the tuna until it is rolled into a cylinder. Apply a little pressure until the roll holds together on its own, then release it from the sheet.
4. Take a sharp knife and slice the roll into approx. 6 pieces.
5. Dot the top of each roll with a bit of Sriracha sauce.

SLICED BELL PEPPERS

- 1 MEDIUM RED BELL PEPPER

1. Wash the bell pepper.
2. Slice it in half, then remove the seeds and stem.
3. Slice into strips and enjoy.

BREAKFAST:

CHIA SEED PAPAYA SHAKE • 1 ¼ CUP ALMOND MILK • 2 TBSP CHIA SEES • ½ CUP CUBED PAPAYA	1. Mix all ingredients in a blender until smooth.
EASY HARD-BOILED EGGS • 1 LARGE EGG	1. Place eggs in a pot: pour water over the eggs to cover. Cover and turn stove to high; bringing to a boil. Turn off heat and place pot on a cool burner for 15 min. 2. Fill a large bowl halfway with cold water; transfer eggs. Chill.

LUNCH:

GRILLED ITALIAN SAUSAGE WITH PEPPERS, ONIONS, AND ARUGULA • ½ TBSP OLIVE OIL • 1 DASH OF SALT • ¾ TBSP BALSAMIC VINEGAR • ½ LARGE RED BELL PEPPER • 1 CUP ARUGULA • ¼ LARGE ONION • ¾ TBSP HONEY • 4 OZ ITALIAN SAUSAGE	1. Preheat grill. Mix together balsamic vinegar and honey into a small bowl; set it aside. 2. Coat onion, pepper, and sausage with olive oil. Add a dash of salt. Coat grill with olive oil. Put onion wedges on grill; cover. Let onions roast for 5 min. Turn onions and move to a cooler part of the grill to finish. 3. If your grill has 2 levels. Place sausage on top part of grill with the peppers below. The sausage juice and fat will drip on the peppers flavoring them. If your grill doesn't have two levels, place peppers on hottest part of grill and sausage on the coolest. 4. Cover and grill for 15-20 min. periodically checking and turning the sausage and peppers. 5. Place on a bed of arugula.
GRILLED POLENTA CHIPS • 2 OZ YELLOW POLENTA • ¼ TBSP OLIVE OIL • ½ TBSP NUTRITIONAL YEAST • 1 DASH OF PEPPER • 1 DASH OF SALT	1. Heat a grill to medium-high heat and rub with olive oil. 2. Cut tube of polenta into ¼ to ½ slices. Brush both sides of polenta cakes with olive oil. Sprinkle both sides with nutritional yeast, salt and pepper. 3. Lay the polenta rounds in one layer on the grill, and grill for 5 minutes on each side or until both sides are golden and crunchy with grill marks. Remove the cakes and place on large plate to cool. 4. Serve warm.

Continued on next page…

ALMONDS

- 1 OZ ALMONDS

1. Enjoy!

DINNER:

EASY GRILLED CHICKEN TERIYAKI

- 8 OZ CHICKEN BREAST
- ¼ CUP TERIYAKI SAUCE
- 1 TBSP LEMON JUICE
- ½ TSP GARLIC
- ½ TSP SESAME OIL

1. Place chicken, teriyaki sauce, lemon juice, garlic, and sesame oil in a large resealable plastic bag. Seal bag and shake to coat.
2. Place in refrigerator for 24 hours. Preheat grill; high. Lightly oil the grill and remove the chicken from the bag, discarding remainder marinade.
3. Grill for 6-8 minutes each side, or until juices run clear when chicken is pierced with a fork.

TOMATO SOUP

- ½ CAN TOMATO SOUP
- ½ CAN WATER

1. Mix together soup and water (using the empty can of soup to measure)
2. Microwave for about 3 minutes.

SNACK:

PROTEIN SALAD

- ½ CAN, DRAINED TUNA
- ½ LARGE EGG
- 1 TBSP MAYONNAISE-LIKE DRESSING
- 1 TBSP LEMON JUICE
- ½ STALK MEDIUM CELERY
- ¼ MEDIUM ONIONS
- .5 OZ SLIVERED ALMONDS

1. Hard boil the egg and chop it into pieces.
2. Chop vegetables.
3. Mix all ingredients including the egg and store in an airtight container.

BANANA

- 1 MEDIUM BANANA

1. Enjoy!

BREAKFAST:

APPLE PIE SMOOTHIE

- ½ CUP ALMOND MILK
- 1 MEDIUM APPLE
- 1.3 OZ PITTED DATES
- .5 OZ GRAMS CHOPPED WALNUTS
- .6 OZ RAISINS
- ½ TSP CINNAMON
- DROP OF VANILLA EXTRACT
- ½ TBSP GROUND FLAXSEED

1. Combine all ingredients in a blender.
2. Pulse until smooth.

BACON

- 2 STRIPS BACON

1. Cook bacon in a skillet over medium to medium-high heat until browned and crisp.
2. Bacon can also be cooked in an oven at 350F for about 20 minutes, or microwave at about 50-60 seconds per strip.

LUNCH:

EASY GRILLED CHICKEN TERIYAKI

- 8 OZ CHICKEN BREAST
- ¼ CUP TERIYAKI SAUCE
- 1 TBSP LEMON JUICE
- ½ TSP GARLIC
- ½ TSP SESAME OIL

1. Place chicken, teriyaki sauce, lemon juice, garlic, and sesame oil in a large resealable plastic bag. Seal bag and shake to coat. Place in refrigerator for 24 hours, turning every so often.
2. Preheat grill for high heat.
3. Lightly oil the grill and remove the chicken from the bag, discarding remainder marinade.
4. Grill for 6-8 minutes each side, or until juices run clear when chicken is pierced with a fork.

ZUCCHINI

- 1 MEDIUM ZUCCHINI

1. Wash zucchini and cut into 2-3-inch chunks.
2. Put through spiralizer or use a peeler.
3. Put in boiling water for about 5 minutes or until they reach the consistency you like.
4. Strain and serve.

Continued on next page…

DINNER:

TURKEY KIELBASA HASH
- 1.7 OZ HASHBROWNS
- 1 SERVING 2 OZ KIELBASA
- 1 TBSP OLIVE OIL
- .6 OZ MEDIUM RED BELL PEPPER
- .3 OZ MEDIUM GREEN BELL PEPPER
- 1 DASH OF SALT
- 1 DASH OF PEPPER
- .6 OZ OF A MEDIUM ONION

1. Cook hash browns according to package directions.
2. In a separate skillet, brown the sliced kielbasa for around 5 minutes in olive oil over medium-high heat. Remove the kielbasa from the pan and set aside. Add the peppers and onions to the skillet and season.
3. Cook for 5 minutes, or until softened, stirring occasionally.
4. Add the cooked hash browns and kielbasa to the skillet with the onions, peppers and mix everything together.
5. Serve hot!

CAULIFLOWER AND TAHINI
- 1 CUP CHOPPED CAULIFLOWER
- 2 TBSP SESAME TAHINI

1. Chop up the cauliflower; retaining some of the florets.
2. Serve cauliflower pieces with tahini for dipping.

SNACK:

PALEO AVOCADO TUNA SALAD
- 1 FRUIT AVOCADO
- 1 LEMON YIELDS LEMON JUICE
- 1 TBSP CHOPPED ONIONS
- 5 OZ OF TUNA
- 1 DASH OF SALT
- 1 DASH OF PEPPER

1. Cut the avocado in half and scoop the middle of both halves into a bowl, leaving a shell of avocado flesh about ¼ inch thick on each side.
2. Add lemon juice, and onion to the avocado in the bowl and mash together. Add drained tune, salt and pepper. Stir to combine all ingredients. (season to liking)
3. Fill avocado shells with tuna salad.

CARROTS
- 1 CUP BABY CARROTS

1. Enjoy!

BREAKFAST:

VEGA ONE BLUEBERRY ACAI SMOOTHIE • ½ CUP WATER • ½ MEDIUM BANANA • ½ TBSP GROUND FLAXSEED • 3 TSP ORGANIC ACAI POWDER • 1 TBSP FLAXSEED OIL • ¾ SERVING, ALL-IN-ONE NUTRITION SHAKE, FRENCH VANILLA • 1 CUP BLUEBERRIES	1. Blend all ingredients in a blender. 2. Pulse until smooth.

LUNCH:

CURRY CHICKEN SALAD • 1 TSP OIL • 4 OZ CHICKEN BREAST • ½ STALK, LARGE CELERY • 4 TSP LIGHT MAYONNAISE • 1/3 TSP CURRY POWDER	1. To cook chicken, first pound out chicken breast a bit to the same thickness by carefully using a kitchen mallet or the back of a heavy jar. 2. Cook in a nonstick pan over medium heat with about a tsp of olive oil (about 4 minutes each side, or until no pink is in the middle) 3. In a medium bowl, stir together the chicken, celery, mayonnaise, and curry powder.
FRIED RIPE PLANTAINS • 1 MEDIUM PLANTAINS • 1 TBSP VEGETABLE OIL • ½ DASH OF SALT	1. Peel the plantains and cut diagonally into ¼ inch thick slices. 2. Drizzle oil into a frying pan just enough to coat the bottom of the pan. 3. Place on medium heat. 4. When oil begins to simmer, add plantains. (work in batches) 5. Fry for 1 ½ minutes on one side then flip and cook for 1 minute on the other side. 6. Remove plantains from pan and rest on paper towels. 7. Continue frying in batches until all the plantains are fried. 8. Sprinkle lightly with salt to give a sweet and salty taste.

Continued on next page…

DINNER:
PORK CHOPS WITH STEWED TOMATOES, CAPERS
AND ROSEMARY

- ¼ TBSP ROSEMARY
- ½ TBSP OLIVE OIL
- ½ CLOVES, MINCED GARLIC
- 6 OZ PORK CENTER RIB (CHOPS)
- ½ TBSP PICKLE RELISH
- ¼ CAN TOMATOES
- ½ TBSP, DRAINED CAPERS

1. Coarsely chop tomatoes in a can with kitchen shears.
2. Pat pork dry, then sprinkle with salt and pepper.
3. Heat oil in a 12-inch heavy skillet over medium-high heat until it simmers. Then brown the chops, turning them once. About 5 minutes total. Transfer pork chops to plate and cover with foil.
4. Keep remaining oil in skillet and sauté garlic over medium-high heat for 30 seconds. Add the tomatoes and remaining ingredients and simmer stirring once or twice, for a total of 3 minutes.
5. Add pork with any remaining juice from the plate, turning to coat, and simmer, uncovered, until just cooked through. 23 minutes. Season with salt and pepper.

GARLIC KALE

- ½ CUP, CHOPPED KALE
- ½ TBSP OLIVE OIL
- 1 CLOVES, MINCED GARLIC

1. Tear the kale leaves into bite-size pieces from the thick stems and discard the stems.
2. Heat the olive oil in a large pot over medium heat. Cook and stir the garlic in the hot oil until softened. (about 2 minutes)
3. Add kale and continue cooking until kale is bright green and wilted. About 5 minutes. Serve.

SNACK:
EASY TOSSED SALAD

- 1 CUP SHREDDED LETTUCE
- 1 MEDIUM WHOLE TOMATO
- 1 LARGE CARROT
- 1 CUCUMBER
- 1 MEDIUM SCALLION
- 1 TBSP RANCH DRESSING

1. Chop the lettuce, tomatoes, carrots, cucumbers, and scallions, then toss it together and add the dressing of your choice.

BANANA

- 1 MEDIUM BANANA

1. Enjoy!

<u>Note</u>: Above is one full day "substitute" meal plan that can be used to interchange any day in Restore week (Tuesday through Friday). Choose this substitute meal plan if you want and substitute it in for any day you choose.

BREAKFAST:

HIGH PROTEIN OMELET	
• 4 LARGE EGG WHITES • 2 LARGE EGG • 2 TSP SALT • 2 TSP PEPPER • 3 TBSP BARBECUE SAUCE	1. Whisk eggs, and salt and pepper to taste. 2. Heat a pan with non-stick spray over medium heat. Pour eggs onto a pan and cook until the egg starts to set. Flip it in half, in the pan and let it sit for another 30 seconds. 3. Add barbecue sauce.

FRUIT SALAD	
• 1 CUP, HALVES OF STRAWBERRIES • 1 CUP BLUEBERRIES	1. Add together in a bowl.

LUNCH:

ZUCCHINI NOODLES WITH MEAT AND MUSHROOM TOMATO SAUCE	
• ½ LARGE ZUCCHINI • ½ TBSP OLIVE OIL • 3 TBSP, CHOPPED ONIONS • 1/3 CUP GARLIC • 2 TBSP DICED MUSHROOM • 3 OZ GROUND TURKEY • 1.7 OZ PLUM TOMATO • 1 TSP TOMATO PASTE • 1 DASH OF SALT • 1 DASH OF PEPPER • 3 TBSP BASIL LEAVES	1. Run 3 large zucchinis through a spiralizer to create noodles. (If you don't have one, you can carefully use a peeler). Set aside. 2. Heat a large saucepan to medium-high heat. 3. Add olive oil and chopped onions to pan. Sauté until translucent. (about 2-3 minutes) 4. Add minced garlic cloves and sauté for 30 seconds and add sliced mushroom. 5. Cook until mushrooms are browned. (about 4-5 minutes) Add ground turkey and sauté until 6. cooked through. (about 6-10 minutes)

DINNER:

PRAWN CURRY	
• ½ TBSP OLIVE OIL • 1 TBSP CURRY PASTE • ½ MEDIUM ONIONS • 7 OZ OF TOMATOES • 3 ½ OZ PRAWNS • ½ CLOVE OF GARLIC • 4 ½ SPRIGS FRESH CILANTRO	1. Drizzle some oil into a large pan and gently heat; then add onions. 2. Sizzle over low-heat for 4 minutes, or until the onions are soft. 3. Stir in the curry paste and cook for a few more minutes. 4. Stir in the prawns and tomatoes, then bring to a simmer. (3-4 minutes or until they are cooked through) 5. Season, and then add the cilantro before serving.

Continued on next page…

GARLIC KALE
- ½ CUP CHOPPED KALE
- ½ TBSP OLIVE OIL
- 1 CLOVE MINCED GARLIC

1. Tear the kale leaves into bite sized pieces from the stems and discard them.
2. Heat the olive oil in a large pot over medium heat. Cook and stir the garlic in the hot oil until softened. (about 2 minutes)
3. Add the kale and continue cooking and stirring until the kale is bright green and wilted, about 5 minutes.

SNACK:

CHICKEN CELERY STICK
- 1 CAN OF CHICKEN
- 2 TBSP MAYONNAISE-LIKE DRESSING
- ½ TSP GARLIC POWDER
- 1 DASH OF SALT
- 3 STALKS LARGE CELERY

1. Combine the chicken, mayo, garlic powder, and salt in a bowl and mix until combined.
2. Cut celery stalks in half. Stuff each stalk with the chicken mixture.

CARROTS
- 1 CUP BABY CARROTS

1. Enjoy!

Note: Above is one full day "substitute" meal plan that can be used to interchange any day in Restore week (Tuesday through Friday). Choose this substitute meal plan if you want and substitute it in for any day you choose.

FOOD ITEM	AVERAGE SERVING SIZE	CALORIES
PROTEIN		
HAMBURGER PATTY	3.5 OZ	235 CAL
TRI TIP	3.5 OZ	182 CAL
PORK CUTLET	3.5 OZ	231 CAL
CHICKEN	4 OZ	190 CAL
BEEF NEW YORK STRIP STEAK	4 OZ	220 CAL
BABY BACK RIBS	3 OZ	270 CAL
PORK SIRLOIN	3 OZ	168 CAL
BEEF RIBEYE STEAK	6 OZ	450 CAL
SALMON	3 OZ	200 CAL
HALIBUT	3 OZ	107 CAL
FRIED EGG	1 LARGE EGG	92 CAL
BOILED EGG	1 LARGE EGG	77 CAL
SCRAMBLED EGG	1 LARGE EGG	101 CAL
CARBOHYDRATES		
BANANA	1 MEDIUM BANANA	104 CAL
APPLE	1 MEDIUM APPLE	80 CAL
ORANGE	1 FRUIT	69 CAL
SPAGHETTI WITH MEAT SAUCE	10 OZ	286 CAL
CHICKEN ALFREDO PASTA	8.14 OZ	321 CAL
WHITE RICE	1 CUP	205 CAL
BROWN RICE	1 CUP	216 CAL
BLACK BEANS	½ CUP	90 CAL
REFRIED BEANS	½ CUP	125 CAL
PINTO BEANS	½ CUP	144 CAL
BROCCOLI	1 CUP	65 CAL
GREEN BEANS	1 CUP	25 CAL
CORN	4 OZ	153 CAL
WHOLE WHEAT BREAD	1 SLICE	69 CAL
WHITE BREAD	1 SLICE	120 CAL
SOURDOUGH BREAD	1 SLICE	120 CAL
RESTAURANTS		

IN N OUT BURGER WITH ONION	1 SERVING	390 CAL
MCDONALDS CHEESEBURGER	1 SERVING	300 CAL
TACO BELL CRUNCHY SUPREME TACO	1 SERVING	190 CAL
TACO BELL BEAN BURRITO	1 SERVING	370 CAL
EL POLLO LOCO AL CARBON CHICKEN TACOS	1 SERVING	160 CAL
JAMBA JUICE ACAI PRIMO FRUIT BOWL	1 SERVING	540 CAL
CARL'S JR SPICY CHICKEN SANDWICH	1 SERVING	460 CAL
SUBWAY HAM SANDWICH 6 INCH	1 SERVING	450 CAL
PANERA BREAD STRAWBERRY POPPYSEED CHICKEN SALAD	1 SERVING	350 CAL
RED LOBSTER STARTER SAMPLER	1 SERVING	620 CAL
OLIVE GARDEN CHICKEN ALFREDO FETTUCCINE	1 SERVING	500 CAL
RED ROBIN WINGS	1 SERVING	1,023 CAL
APPLEBEE'S TRIPLE BACON BURGER	1 SERVING	1,190 CAL

Note: Above is an example of some but not all food items allowed in Combo. Remember you can eat anything you want in Combo (Saturday and Sunday) as long as you stay within your targeted caloric intake.

RECIPE: COMBO   *SATURDAY- SUNDAY: 1,800 CALORIES*

SATURDAY BREAKFAST:

- 3 WAFFLES
  (278 CALORIES)
- 2 EGGS
  (140 CALORIES)
- 4 TBSP LITE SYRUP
  (105 CALORIES)

SATURDAY LUNCH:

- 1 PANERA GRILLED CHICKEN CAESAR SALAD
  (400 CALORIES)
- 4 TBSP HIDDEN VALLEY RANCH DRESSING
  (220 CALORIES)

SATURDAY DINNER:

- 4 OZ TRI TIP
  (171 CALORIES)
- 1 BAKED POTATO
  (145 CALORIES)
- 1 CUP MIXED VEGGIES (20 CALORIES)

SATURDAY SNACK:

- JAMBA JUICE STRAWBERRY WILD
  (370 CALORIES)

TOTAL: 1,849 CALORIES

SUNDAY BREAKFAST:

- 2 EGGS
  (140 CALORIES)
- 1 CUP HASHBROWN POTATOES
  (413 CALORIES)
- 1 OZ PORK CHORIZO (49 CALORIES)

SUNDAY LUNCH:

- 1 IN N OUT HAMBURGER (390 CALORIES)
- 1 SMALL FRY
  (230 CALORIES)

SUNDAY DINNER:

- 1 CUP MEAT LOAF
  (660 CALORIES)

TOTAL: 1,882 CALORIES

Note: In Combo you can eat ANY food, but stay in your caloric intake!

Macro Circuit Recipe

2,000 Calorie Meal Plan

These meal plans are for those people who have the extra time to cook meals with recipes.

MONDAY BREAKFAST: (EXAMPLE 1)	MONDAY BREAKFAST: (EXAMPLE 2)
HOT BROTH • 12 OZ BEEF BROTH, HEATED	ORANGE JUICE • 12 OZ ORANGE JUICE (NO PULP)
LUNCH:	LUNCH:
APPLE JUICE • 12 OZ APPLE JUICE	GRAPE JUICE • 12 OZ GRAPE JUICE
DINNER:	DINNER:
CRANBERRY JUICE • 12 OZ CRANBERRY JUICE	TOMATO JUICE • 12 OZ TOMATO JUICE
SNACK:	SNACK:
WATER • 12 OZ WATER	VEGETABLE JUICE • 12 OZ VEGETABLE JUICE

<u>Reminder:</u> These are 2 examples of what your Mondays will look like. DO NOT FOLLOW THIS PLAN.

Things You Can Have During Your Flush: (Calories for 8 fl ounces)

- Coconut Water (46 Calories)
- Water (0 Calories)
- Carrot Juice (94 Calories)
- Apple Juice (105 Calories)
- Orange Juice (115 Calories)
- Grape Juice (152 Calories)
- Vegetable Juice (50 Calories)
- Pomegranate Juice (140 Calories)
- Tomato Juice (41 Calories)
- Grapefruit Juice (102 Calories)
- Cranberry Juice (116 Calories)
- Chicken Broth (41 Calories)
- Beef Broth (10 Calories)
- Tea (nothing added) (2.4 Calories)
- Coffee (nothing added) (1.8 Calories)

Note: This is a 24-hour fast. No food is to be consumed during this time. It is advised to only choose from the options above. Stay within your caloric intake. This meal plan is just an EXAMPLE of what your Mondays should look like.

BREAKFAST:

| PINEAPPLE COCONUT VITAMIN C SMOOTHIE | 1. Place all ingredients in a blender and puree until smooth. Pour into a glass and serve. |

PINEAPPLE COCONUT VITAMIN C SMOOTHIE
- 1 CUP PINEAPPLE CHUNKS
- 1 MEDIUM BANANA
- 1 CUP UNSWEETENED COCONUT MILK
- ½ CUP ORANGE JUICE

1. Place all ingredients in a blender and puree until smooth. Pour into a glass and serve.

EASY HARD-BOILED EGGS
- 2 LARGE EGGS

1. Place eggs in a pot; pour enough water over eggs to cover. Cover and turn stove to high; bring to boil; turn off heat and place pot on a cool burner.
2. Let the pot sit with the cover on for 15 minutes. Fill a large bowl halfway with cold water, transfer the eggs from the pot to the cold water.
3. Replace the water with cold water as needed to keep cold until the eggs are completely cooled. Chill in refrigerator.

LUNCH:

TACO SALAD
- 8 OZ GROUND BEEF
- 3 CUP SPINACH
- 1/3 CUP CHOPPED ONION
- ¼ CUP CHOPPED RED BELL PEPPER
- ¼ CUP SALSA

1. Cook ground beef in a pan until evenly browned through and no longer pink.
2. Chop up greens and veggies and combine in a bowl.
3. Add the beef; mix well. Add salsa as a light dressing, mix well, serve and enjoy.

SLICED BELL PEPPER
- 1 MEDIUM RED BELL PEPPER

1. Wash the bell pepper, slice in half, remove the seeds and stem. Slice into strips and enjoy!

DINNER:

PINEAPPLE SHRIMP SALAD
- 4 OZ. SHRIMP
- ½ TBSP. OLIVE OIL
- 1 SMALL ONION
- ½ PINEAPPLE CHUNKS
- ½ SMALL RED BELL PEPPER
- ½ FRUIT AVOCADO
- 1 LIME YIELDS JUICE
- 1 CUP SHREDDED LETTUCE

1. Cook the shrimp with olive oil, salt and pepper over medium heat until bright pink and cooked through.
2. Toss together with remaining ingredients.

Continued on next page…

KALE CHIPS

- 2 CUPS CHOPPED KALE
- ½ TBSP OLIVE OIL
- ½ TSP SALT

1. Preheat oven to 350 degrees.
2. Remove the center ribs and stems from kale if present.
3. Tear kale leaves into 3-4-inch pieces.
4. Toss kale leaves in olive oil and salt. Spread on baking sheet coated with cooking spray. Bake for 12-15 minutes at 350 degrees until browned around edges and crisp.

SNACK:

LIME CHICKEN SALAD

- 1 CAN OF CHICKEN
- 2 TSP LIME JUICE
- 1 DASH OF SALT
- 4 LARGE LETTUCE LEAVES

1. Combine the chicken, lime juice, and salt.
2. Arrange the bib lettuce leaves and serve the chicken salad on top.

CAULIFLOWER AND TAHINI

- 1 CUP CHOPPED CAULIFLOWER
- 2 TBSP SESAME TAHINI

1. Chop the cauliflower lovingly, to retain some of the florets.
2. Serve cauliflower pieces with tahini for dipping.

BREAKFAST:

PROTEIN SOUTHWEST SCRAMBLE
- 4 LARGE EGG WHITES
- ½ SAUSAGE LINK
- 2 TSP OLIVE OIL
- 1 MEDIUM ONION
- ½ CUP CHOPPED RED BELL PEPPER
- 1 CUP SPINACH
- 1 MEDIUM WHOLE TOMATO
- 1 DASH OF SALT
- 1 DASH OF PEPPER

1. Dice the tomato, chop the red pepper, onion, and turkey sausage.
2. In a large pan, drizzle the onions and peppers with olive oil and sauté.
3. When the onions are clear and peppers are tender, season with salt and pepper.
4. Add chopped turkey sausage, and sauté until sausage is golden brown. Lower heat, add egg whites, and scramble. When eggs are almost done, add in tomato and spinach, mix around, and then serve.

GRILLED PEACHES WITH HONEY
- ½ MEDIUM PEACH
- 5 TSP OLIVE OIL
- DRIP OF HONEY

1. Preheat grill to high. Cut peaches in half, remove pits.
2. Brush cut side of peach halves with olive oil and place on grill, cut side down.
3. Grill until golden brown and caramelized, 2-3 minutes.
4. Turn peach halves over and grill until slightly soft and warmed through, about 2 minutes longer.
5. Remove from grill and drizzle with honey.

LUNCH:

KIELBASA AND CAULIFLOWER STIR-FRY
- ¼ TBSP OLIVE OIL
- 8 OZ KIELBASA
- ¼ HEAD LARGE CAULIFLOWER
- ¼ CUP ONIONS
- 1 DASH OF PEPPER
- ½ CLOVE MINCED GARLIC

1. Heat olive oil in large skillet over medium-high heat.
2. Add kielbasa and cook until well browned, about 6 minutes. Remove from skillet and set aside on a plate. Reserve pan drippings.
3. In pan drippings, add the cauliflower florets, cover and cook for 5 minutes.
4. Add onion, stir, and cook 5 minutes. Keep covered.
5. Add the garlic, keep uncovered and cook 1 additional minute.
6. Return the kielbasa to the pan and heat through.

Continued on next page…

FRIED PLANTAINS
- ¼ MEDIUM PLANTAIN
- 3 TSP VEGETABLE OIL
- ¼ TSP CHILI POWDER

1. Preheat oil in a large, deep skillet over medium high heat. Peel the plantains and cut them in half. Slice the halves lengthwise into thin pieces.
2. Fry the pieces until browned and tender. Drain the excess oil on paper towels. Sprinkle with chili powder.

DINNER:

BAKED COCONUT CILANTRO TILAPIA
- 5 OZ TILAPIA
- 1 CUP COCONUT MILK
- 1 DASH FRESH CILANTRO
- .3 OZ WATER
- ½ CLOVE MINCED GARLIC
- 1 DASH PEPPER
- 1 DASH CAYENNE PEPPER
- 1 DASH GROUND CUMIN
- 1 DASH CURRY POWDER
- 1 DASH OF SALT
- 1 SPRAY OF PAM COOKING SPRAY

1. Preheat oven to 425 degrees. Lightly spray a baking dish with cooking spray.
2. Wash fillets and pat dry. Place fish in baking dish and set aside.
3. Combine remaining ingredients in a bowl and whisk well. Evenly pour mixture over fish.
4. Bake fish for about 15 minutes until opaque in center.
5. Serve with your choice of rice or another side dish.

CARROTS
- 1 CUP BABY CARROTS

1. Enjoy alone or with hummus on the side.

SNACK:

HEMP PROTEIN SHAKE
- 1 SERVING MANITOBA HEMP PROTEIN POWDER
- 1 TBSP RAW AGAVE NECTAR
- 1 TBSP CINNAMON
- ½ SERVING LIVING HARVEST HEMP MILK
- 1 MEDIUM BANANA
- ½ CUP WATER

1. Combine all ingredients in a blender and pulse until smooth.

SLICED BELL PEPPER
- 1 MEDIUM RED BELL PEPPER

1. Wash the bell pepper, slice it in half, remove seeds and stem. Slice into strips.

BREAKFAST:

HIGH PROTEIN OMELET
- 4 LARGE EGG WHITES
- 2 LARGE EGGS
- 2 TSP SALT
- 2 TSP PEPPER
- 3 TBSP BARBECUE SAUCE

1. Whisk eggs, add salt and pepper to taste. Heat a pan with nonstick spray over medium heat.
2. Pour eggs onto pan and cook until most of the egg is turning solid.
3. Fold in half in pan and let sit for 30 seconds.
4. Add barbecue sauce for taste.

BACON
- 2 SLICES BACON

1. Cook bacon in a skillet over medium to medium-high heat until browned and crisp, turning to brown evenly.
2. Bacon can also be cooked in an oven at 350 degrees for about 20 minutes, or microwave at about 50-60 seconds per strip.

LUNCH:

ROSEMARY LEMON GRILLED SCALLOPS
- 1 TBSP ROSEMARY
- 9 OZ SCALLOPS
- ½ TBSP OLIVE OIL
- 1 DASH OF SALT
- 1 DASH OF PEPPER
- ½ LEMON YIELDS LEMON JUICE

1. Preheat grill to medium-high.
2. Pluck leaves from center of rosemary sprig, leaving leaves on both ends. Chop leaves finely.
3. Skewer scallops on center of rosemary sprig. Rub scallops with olive oil, sprinkle on chopped rosemary, and salt and pepper to taste.
4. Grill on medium high for 3-4 minutes per side. Grill ½ lemon at the same time. Remove from the grill and serve with the lemon wedge.

DINNER:

GRILLED PINEAPPLE WITH CINNAMON HONEY DRIZZLE
- 5 OZ PINEAPPLE
- 2 TBSP HONEY
- 1 DASH CINNAMON

1. Grill pineapple slices over medium heat for 510 minutes.
2. While the pineapple is grilling, mix together the honey (softened in the microwave for about 30 seconds) and the cinnamon.
3. Drizzle the grilled pineapple with the honey and serve.

CAULIFLOWER AND TAHINI
- 1 CUP CHOPPED CAULIFLOWER
- 2 TBSP SESAME TAHINI

1. Chop the cauliflower lovingly, to retain some of the florets.
2. Serve the cauliflower pieces with tahini for dipping.

Continued on next page…

AVOCADO AND VEGGIE SALAD
- 2 CUP SHREDDED LETTUCE
- ½ CUP CHOPPED OR SLICED TOMATOES
- 2 MEDIUM RADISHES
- ½ CUP CHOPPED CUCUMBER
- ½ CUP SLICED GREEN BELL PEPPER
- 1 FRUIT AVOCADO
- ¼ TSP PEPPER OR HOT SAUCE
- 2 TSP MAYO-LIKE DRESSING
- 1 LIME YIELDS JUICE

1. Gently toss the veggies in a bowl, excluding avocado.
2. Mash the avocado with hot sauce, mayo, and half the lime juice.
3. Squeeze remaining lime juice over salad and top with avocado mixture.

ALMONDS
- 1 OZ ALMONDS

1. Enjoy!

CARROTS
- 1 CUP BABY CARROTS

1. Enjoy by themselves. Optionally, enjoy with a side of hummus.

BREAKFAST:

ONION AND TOMATO OMELET
- 2 EXTRA LARGE EGGS
- 2 TBSP CHOPPED ONIONS
- 1 DASH OF SALT
- ¼ CUP CHOPPED OR SLICED TOMATOES
- 1 TBSP VEGETABLE OIL

1. Scramble eggs in a bowl. Set aside.
2. Heat oil in skillet, add tomatoes and onions. Cook until soft.
3. Add eggs to skillet and begin to swirl until eggs are set. Season with salt. Fold
4. one side of omelet over and remove from pan.

LUNCH:

QUICK AND SIMPLE STIR-FRIED KALE AND BACON
- 20 OZ KALE
- 12 STRIPS COOKED BACON
- 1 DASH SALT
- 1 DASH PEPPER
- 2 LEMONS WITHOUT SEEDS

1. Wash and chop kale leaves and prep remaining ingredients.
2. Sauté the bacon bits in a large cast iron skillet over medium heat. Once they are crisp, add in kale leaves with a dash of salt and pepper.
3. Stir the kale and bacon for a couple minutes and then splash on some lemon juice.

BALSAMIC ASPARAGUS
- 12 LARGE SPEARS, ASPARAGUS
- ½ TBSP OLIVE OIL
- 1 DASH OF PEPPER
- ½ TBSP BALSAMIC VINEGAR

1. Prepare asparagus by washing and snapping off tough ends.
2. Heat oil in frying pan.
3. Add asparagus and keep moving around in pan until changes color. (approx. 3-5 minutes) add balsamic vinegar and pepper sprinkling over all of the asparagus.
4. Remove from heat and cover for a few minutes to let flavors develop.
5. Serve.

DINNER:

PINEAPPLE, MANGO, AND SPINACH SMOOTHIE
- 1 CUP SPINACH
- 1 CUP PINEAPPLE
- 1 CUP MANGO
- 1 SMALL BANANA
- 1 CUP WATER

1. Combine all ingredients in blender and pulse until smooth.

ZUCCHINI SPEARS
- 9 ZUCCHINI
- 1 DASH OF SALT

1. Cut zucchini lengthwise and cut into ¼" wedges.
2. Cook zucchini in boiling salted water until crisp-tender, about 1 minute. Drain and sprinkle with salt.

Continued on next page…

SNACK:

CLASSIC TUNA SALAD
- 1 CAN TUNA
- 1 TSP DIJON MUSTARD
- ¼ CUP MAYO-LIKE DRESSING
- 1 TBSP PARSLEY
- 1 DASH OF PEPPER
- ¼ TSP SALT
- ¼ CLOVE, MINCED GARLIC
- .3 OZ PICKLES
- 1 TBSP LEMON JUICE
- ½ STALK CELERY
- 1 TBSP CHOPPED ONION

1. Place the tuna in a colander and drain well.
2. Shred the tuna with your fingers, breaking up any chunks, and creating an even texture.
3. Put tuna in a medium bowl and mix with lemon juice, celery, onion, pickle, garlic, salt, pepper, and parsley, until well blended. Fold in mayo and Dijon until mixture is
4. evenly moistened.

BREAKFAST:

EGGS IN SPICY TOMATO SAUCE

- ½ TBSP OLIVE OIL
- ½ MEDIUM RED BELL PEPPER
- ½ JALAPENO PEPPER
- ¼ ONION
- 1 TSP GARLIC, MINCED
- ½ TSP GROUND CUMIN
- 1 DASH OF SALT
- .4 OZ TOMATO PASTE
- 7 OZ TOMATO
- 2 TBSP WATER
- 2 EXTRA LARGE EGGS
- ½ TBSP PARSLEY

1. Remove seeds from bell peppers and chop.
2. Chop jalapenos and set aside.
3. Heat oil in skillet over medium heat. Add bell peppers, jalapenos, onions, garlic, cumin, and dash of the salt. Cook while stirring occasionally, until the onion becomes translucent, about 7 minutes.
4. Add the tomato paste, mix well.
5. Add canned tomatoes and their liquid, plus 2 tbsp. of water. Bring the mixture to a low boil. Simmer for about 7 minutes, stir occasionally, until sauce has thickened.
6. Using the back of a large spoon, make divots in the tomato sauce for the eggs. Carefully crack each egg into each space. Do not stir.
7. Cover skillet and simmer for about 8 minutes or until eggs are done to your liking. Sprinkle eggs with remaining salt, freshly ground pepper, and chopped fresh cilantro.

PECANS ·

  1 OZ PECANS

1. Enjoy!

LUNCH:

PINEAPPLE, MANGO, AND SPINACH SMOOTHIE

- 1 CUP SPINACH
- 1 CUP PINEAPPLE
- 1 CUP MANGO
- 1 SMALL BANANA
- 1 CUP WATER

1. Combine all ingredients in blender and pulse until smooth.

Continued on next page…

GRILLED ASPARAGUS
- ½ LB ASPARAGUS
- ½ TBSP OLIVE OIL
- ½ DASH SALT
- ½ DASH PEPPER

1. Heat grill to medium
2. Coat asparagus with olive oil and season with salt and pepper.
3. Grill for 2-3 minutes or until tender.

CHICKEN STRIPS
- 2 OZ BONELESS SKINLESS CHICKEN BREAST
- ¼ TSP OLIVE OIL
- ½ DASH SALT
- ½ DASH PEPPER

1. Preheat oven to 400 degrees.
2. Slice the breasts into two then cut into diagonal strips.
3. Put some foil on top of the baking tray. Cover it with a thin layer of olive oil and place some chicken strips on top.
4. Season and turn the strips over, so both sides have olive oil on them.
5. Bake at the top of the oven for 10 minutes, then flip them over and bake for another 5.
6. Serve hot.

DINNER:

INDIAN FLAVORED POUNDED CHICKEN
- ½ TSP GROUND CUMIN
- ½ TSP TURMERIC
- ½ TSP CORIANDER LEAF
- ½ TSP ONION POWDER
- 1 DASH OF SALT
- 1 DASH OF PEPPER
- 1 TSP OLIVE OIL
- 4 OZ BONELESS SKINLESS CHICKEN BREAST

1. In a small bowl, combine ground cumin, turmeric, ground coriander, onion powder, salt, black pepper, and olive oil, set aside. Starting at the thicker side using a sharp knife make a lengthwise horizontal cut into the top 2/3 of the chicken breast stopping before cutting all the way through. Fold the chicken breast open like a book (it should still be in one piece)
2. Put it between 2 pieces of plastic wrap and pound it out on both sides with the flat side of a meat tenderizer working from the center out until it spreads to double its original size and about ¼ inch thick.
3. Remove plastic wrap and rub the olive-spice paste evenly across one side of the chicken.
4. Cover with plastic wrap and lightly pound in the seasoning with the toothy side of the meat tenderizer. Flip the breast, rub the remaining olive- spice into the other side of the chicken breast, cover with plastic wrap and lightly pound in the seasoning.
5. Heat olive oil in a large pan over high heat, when it's sizzling, add the chicken breast. Put a weight on it, cook for one minute, then flip, add the weight and cook for another one minute.
6. Transfer to a plate and let it rest for 3 minutes. Serve hot and enjoy!

Continued on next page…

EASY GRILLED PEPPERS
- 3/4 LARGE RED BELL PEPPER
- ½ TBSP OLIVE OIL
- 1 DASH OF SALT
- 1 DASH OF PEPPER
- 0.3 OZ PARSLEY

1. Prepare outdoor grill for covered direct grilling on medium.
2. Cut peppers lengthwise into quarters. Discard stems and seeds.
3. Toss peppers with oil, salt, and pepper. Place on grill and cook and cover for 4-5 minutes.
4. Flip over and cook for an additional 3-4 minutes. Add parsley and toss together.

SNACK:

KALE AVOCADO SALAD
- 2 CUPS CHOPPED KALE
- 1 FRUIT AVOCADO
- ½ LEMON WITHOUT SEEDS
- 2 TSP PEPPER
- 1 TSP SALT

1. Chop kale.
2. Mash avocado into kale.
3. Add lemon or lime juice.
4. Salt and pepper to taste.
5. Toss and enjoy!

BANANA
- 1 MEDIUM BANANA

1. Enjoy!

Note: Above is one full day "substitute" meal plan that can be used to interchange any day in Restore week (Tuesday through Friday). Choose this substitute meal plan if you want and substitute it in for any day you choose.

BREAKFAST:

ANTIOXIDANT SMOOTHIE
- 2 CUP SPINACH
- 2 CUP SHREDDED LETTUCE
- ½ POMEGRANATE
- ½ UNTHAWED BLUEBERRIES
- ½ UNTHAWED STRAWBERRIES
- 2 PITTED DATES
- 1 TBSP. GROUND FLAXSEED
- ¼ FRUIT AVOCADO

1. Combine all ingredients in a blender and pulse until smooth. Add water, as needed.

EASY HARD-BOILED EGGS
- 2 LARGE EGGS

1. Place eggs in a pot; pour enough water over the eggs to cover. Cover and turn the stove on high to bring water to a boil; turn off the heat and place the pot on a cool burner.
2. Let the pot sit covered for 15 minutes. Meanwhile, fill a bowl halfway with cold water. Transfer eggs from the pot to the cold water.
3. Replace the water with cold water as needed to keep cold until the eggs are totally cooled.

LUNCH:

TACO SALAD
- 8 OZ GROUND BEEF
- 3 CUP SPINACH
- 1/3 CUP CHOPPED ONIONS
- ¼ CUP CHOPPED RED BELL PEPPER
- ¼ CUP SALSA

1. Cook ground beef in a pan until evenly browned through and no longer pink.
2. Chop up greens and veggies and combine in a bowl. Add the beef; mix well. Add the salsa as a light dressing.
3. Mix well and serve.

ROASTED CHERRY TOMATOES WITH MINT
- ½ TBSP SPEARMINT
- 1 DASH OF SALT
- 1 DASH OF PEPPER
- 1 TSP OLIVE OIL
- ½ CUP CHERRY TOMATOES

1. Finely chop mint.
2. Preheat oven to 425 degrees.
3. Toss tomatoes with oil, salt, and pepper in a small baking sheet and roast in the middle of the oven, until skins just begin to split, 5-10 minutes.
4. Sprinkle tomatoes with mint.

Continued on next page…

LEMON STEAMED BROCCOLI

- 6 OZ BROCCOLI
- ¼ TSP SALT
- ¼ TSP PEPPER
- ¼ TBSP OLIVE OIL
- 1 TSP LEMON JUICE

1. Trim the broccoli into large florets. Place the broccoli in a steaming basket over boiling water; cover and steam for 3 minutes.
2. Remove lid for a moment, then cook, partially covered, until stems are tender firm, another 8-10 minutes.
3. Remove to platter, season with salt and pepper. Olive oil, and lemon juice.

DINNER:

PORK CHOPS WITH STEWED TOMATOES, CAPERS, AND ROSEMARY

- 1 DASH ROSEMARY
- ½ TBSP OLIVE OIL
- ½ CLOVE, MINCED GARLIC
- 6 OZ PORK CENTER RIB CHOPS
- ½ TBSP PICKLE RELISH
- ¼ CAN TOMATOES
- ½ TBSP DRAINED CAPERS

1. Coarsely chop tomatoes in can with kitchen shears.
2. Pat pork dry, then sprinkle with salt and pepper.
3. Heat oil in 12-inch heavy skillet over medium-high heat until it shimmers, then brown chops, turning once, about 5 minutes total. Transfer to plate and cover with foil.
4. Add remaining oil to skillet and sauté garlic over medium-high heat 30 seconds. Add tomatoes and remaining ingredients and simmer, stirring once or twice, 3 minutes.
5. Add pork with any juices from plate, turning to coat, and simmer, uncovered, until just cooked through, 2-3 minutes. Season with salt and pepper.

ZUCCHINI SPEARS

- 9 OZ ZUCCHINI
- 1 DASH OF SALT

1. Cut zucchini lengthwise and cut into ¼ inch wedges.
2. Cook zucchini in boiling water until crisp tender, about 1 minute. Drain and sprinkle with salt.

Continued on next page…

TURKEY SALAD
- 1 CUP CHOPPED OR DICED TURKEY
- 1 CUP SHREDDED LETTUCE
- 1 TBSP MAYO-LIKE DRESSING
- 1 SERVING TABLE BLEND SALT FREE SEASONING BLEND
- 1 DASH SALT
- 1 DASH PEPPER
- 1 TSP LEMON JUICE

1. Put seasonings, lemon juice, turkey, and mayo in a bowl. Mix well. Serve on top of lettuce.

CINNAMON APPLE BITES
- 1 MEDIUM APPLE
- 1 TSP CINNAMON

1. Cut up apple into bite sized pieces.
2. Put the chopped apple into a container with a lid.
3. Sprinkle on the cinnamon, put the lid on the container, and gently shake.
4. Eat and enjoy immediately.

<u>Note:</u> Above is one full day "substitute" meal plan that can be used to interchange any day in Restore week (Tuesday through Friday). Choose this substitute meal plan if you want and substitute it in for any day you choose.

FOOD ITEM	AVERAGE SERVING SIZE	CALORIES
PROTEIN		
HAMBURGER PATTY	3.5 OZ	235 CAL
TRI TIP	3.5 OZ	182 CAL
PORK CUTLET	3.5 OZ	231 CAL
CHICKEN	4 OZ	190 CAL
BEEF NEW YORK STRIP STEAK	4 OZ	220 CAL
BABY BACK RIBS	3 OZ	270 CAL
PORK SIRLOIN	3 OZ	168 CAL
BEEF RIBEYE STEAK	6 OZ	450 CAL
SALMON	3 OZ	200 CAL
HALIBUT	3 OZ	107 CAL
FRIED EGG	1 LARGE EGG	92 CAL
BOILED EGG	1 LARGE EGG	77 CAL
SCRAMBLED EGG	1 LARGE EGG	101 CAL
CARBOHYDRATES		
BANANA	1 MEDIUM BANANA	104 CAL
APPLE	1 MEDIUM APPLE	80 CAL
ORANGE	1 FRUIT	69 CAL
SPAGHETTI WITH MEAT SAUCE	10 OZ	286 CAL
CHICKEN ALFREDO PASTA	8.14 OZ	321 CAL
WHITE RICE	1 CUP	205 CAL
BROWN RICE	1 CUP	216 CAL
BLACK BEANS	½ CUP	90 CAL
REFRIED BEANS	½ CUP	125 CAL
PINTO BEANS	½ CUP	144 CAL
BROCCOLI	1 CUP	65 CAL
GREEN BEANS	1 CUP	25 CAL
CORN	4 OZ	153 CAL
WHOLE WHEAT BREAD	1 SLICE	69 CAL
WHITE BREAD	1 SLICE	120 CAL
SOURDOUGH BREAD	1 SLICE	120 CAL
RESTAURANTS		

IN N OUT BURGER WITH ONION	1 SERVING	390 CAL
MCDONALDS CHEESEBURGER	1 SERVING	300 CAL
TACO BELL CRUNCHY SUPREME TACO	1 SERVING	190 CAL
TACO BELL BEAN BURRITO	1 SERVING	370 CAL
EL POLLO LOCO AL CARBON CHICKEN TACOS	1 SERVING	160 CAL
JAMBA JUICE ACAI PRIMO FRUIT BOWL	1 SERVING	540 CAL
CARL'S JR SPICY CHICKEN SANDWICH	1 SERVING	460 CAL
SUBWAY HAM SANDWICH 6 INCH	1 SERVING	450 CAL
PANERA BREAD STRAWBERRY POPPYSEED CHICKEN SALAD	1 SERVING	350 CAL
RED LOBSTER STARTER SAMPLER	1 SERVING	620 CAL
OLIVE GARDEN CHICKEN ALFREDO FETTUCCINE	1 SERVING	500 CAL
RED ROBIN WINGS	1 SERVING	1,023 CAL
APPLEBEE'S TRIPLE BACON BURGER	1 SERVING	1,190 CAL

<u>Note:</u> Above is an example of some but not all food items allowed in Combo. Remember you can eat anything you want in Combo (Saturday and Sunday)

SATURDAY BREAKFAST:

- 2 IHOP EGGS (140 CALORIES)
- 1 SERVING IHOP HASHBROWNS (224 CALORIES)
- 1 IHOP BACON (40 CALORIES)
- 1 IHOP PANCAKE (157 CALORIES)
- .5 OZ IHOP SYRUP (55 CALORIES)

SATURDAY LUNCH:

- TUNA MELT (408 CALORIES)
- 1 CHEETO SNACK BAG (160 CALORIES)

SATURDAY DINNER:

- 1 PERSONAL PIZZA (850 CALORIES)

SATURDAY SNACK:

- JAMBA JUICE STRAWBERRY WILD (370 CALORIES)

TOTAL: 2,033 CALORIES

SUNDAY BREAKFAST:

- 1.5 CUPS LUCKY CHARMS CEREAL (220 CALORIES)
- 1 CUP MILK (108 CALORIES)

SUNDAY LUNCH:

- 10 BBQ WINGS (880 CALORIES)
- 8 FL OZ SODA (119 CALORIES)

SUNDAY DINNER:

- 4 OZ CHICKEN (253 CALORIES)
- 1 CUP SUPER SWEET CORN (120 CALORIES)
- 1 BEER (306 CALORIES)

TOTAL: 2,007 CALORIES

<u>Note:</u> In Combo you can eat ANY food, but stay in your caloric intake!

<u>Macro Circuit Recipe</u>

2,500 Calorie Meal Plan

These meal plans are for those people who have the extra time to cook meals with recipes.

RECIPE: FLUSH   *MONDAY: 2,500 CALORIES*

MONDAY BREAKFAST: (EXAMPLE 1)	MONDAY BREAKFAST: (EXAMPLE 2)
HOT BROTH • 12 OZ BEEF BROTH, HEATED	ORANGE JUICE • 12 OZ ORANGE JUICE (NO PULP)
LUNCH:	LUNCH:
APPLE JUICE • 12 OZ APPLE JUICE	GRAPE JUICE • 12 OZ GRAPE FRUIT
DINNER:	DINNER:
CRANBERRY JUICE • 12 OZ CRANBERRY JUICE	TOMATO JUICE • 12 OZ TOMATO JUICE
SNACK:	SNACK:
WATER • 12 OZ WATER	VEGETABLE JUICE • 12 OZ VEGETABLE JUICE

<u>Reminder:</u> These are 2 examples of what your Mondays will look like. DO NOT FOLLOW THIS PLAN.

Things You Can Have During Your Flush: (Calories for 8 fl ounces)

- Coconut Water (46 Calories)
- Water (0 Calories)
- Carrot Juice (94 Calories)
- Apple Juice (105 Calories)
- Orange Juice (115 Calories)
- Grape Juice (152 Calories)
- Vegetable Juice (50 Calories)
- Pomegranate Juice (140 Calories)
- Tomato Juice (41 Calories)
- Grapefruit Juice (102 Calories)
- Cranberry Juice (116 Calories)
- Chicken Broth (41 Calories)
- Beef Broth (10 Calories)
- Tea (nothing added) (2.4 Calories)
- Coffee (nothing added) (1.8 Calories)

Note: This is a 24 hour-fast. No food is to be consumed during this time. It is advised to only choose from the options above. Stay within your caloric intake. This meal plan is just an EXAMPLE of what your Mondays should look like.

BREAKFAST:

ENGLISH MUFFIN EGG SANDWICH

- ½ TBSP OLIVE OIL
- 2 ENGLISH MUFFINS
- 2 LARGE EGGS
- ½ FRUIT AVOCADO
- ¼ TSP GARLIC POWDER
- ¼ TSP CAYENNE PEPPER

1. Place skillet over medium heat and add olive oil, heating for about 5 minutes.
2. Place muffin in toaster oven on toast setting.
3. Crack egg into pan, cooking for 3 minutes and flipping to cook 1 minute on the opposite side. Season with salt and pepper if desired.
4. Remove muffin from toaster and place egg on bottom slice. Add sliced avocado and season with garlic powder and cayenne.
5. Add top slice of muffin and enjoy!

FRUIT SALAD

- 1 CUP HALVED STRAWBERRIES
- 1 CUP BLUEBERRIES

1. Enjoy!

LUNCH:

BALSAMIC CHICKEN AND MUSHROOM

- ½ TSP VEGETABLE OIL
- 7 OZ BALSAMIC VINEGAR
- ½ TSP DIJON MUSTARD
- ¼ CLOVES, MINCED GARLIC
- 4 OZ BONELESS SKINLESS CHICKEN BREAST
- ½ CUP SLICED MUSHROOMS
- .7 OZ CHICKEN BROTH
- 1 DASH THYME

1. In a nonstick skillet, heat vegetable oil.
2. In a bowl mix vinegar, mustard, and garlic. Add chicken and coat both sides with the mixture. Transfer the chicken and mixture to the skillet; sauté until cooked through, about 3 minutes per side. Transfer to a plate and keep warm.
3. In the skillet, heat remaining oil. Sauté the mushrooms about a minute; add broth, thyme, and remaining vinegar. Cook, stirring frequently until the mushrooms are deep brown, about 2 minutes longer.
4. Serve the chicken topped with mushrooms.

BALSAMIC SAUTEED SPINACH

- 2 TBSP OLIVE OIL
- 4 CUP SPINACH
- 4 TBSP BALSAMIC VINEGAR
- .1 DASH SALT
- 1 DASH PEPPER

1. Heat olive oil in a pan over medium-high heat. Cook spinach in olive oil and add balsamic
2. vinegar, salt, and pepper. Let spinach heat through and cook until
3. slightly wilted. Remove from heat and enjoy.

Continued on next page…

DINNER:

BALSAMIC RED WINE GLAZED FILET MIGNON

- 8 OZ BEEF TENDERLOIN
- ½ TSP PEPPER
- 1 TSP SALT
- ¼ CUP BALSAMIC VINEGAR
- 2 FL OZ RED WINE

1. Sprinkle freshly ground pepper over both sides of steak, and sprinkle with salt to taste.
2. Heat a nonstick skillet over medium-high heat. Place steaks in hot pan, and cook for one minute on each side, or until browned.
3. Reduce heat to medium-low and add balsamic vinegar and red wine.
4. Cover, and cook for 4 minutes on each side, basting with sauce when you turn the meat over.
5. Remove steak to warmed plate, spoon tablespoon of glaze over each, serve immediately.

EASY GRILLED PEPPERS

- 3/4 LARGE RED BELL PEPPER
- ½ TBSP OLIVE OIL
- 1 DASH OF SALT
- 1 DASH OF PEPPER
- .3 OZ PARSLEY

1. Prepare outdoor grill for covered direct grilling on medium.
2. Cut each pepper lengthwise into quarters; discard stems and seeds. In medium bowl, toss peppers with oil, salt, and pepper. Place peppers skin side up, on hot grill rack. Cover
3. grill and cook peppers 4-5 minutes or until beginning to soften. Turn peppers over, cover and cook for 3-4 minutes longer or until slightly charred. As peppers are done, return to same bowl. Add parsley and toss to coat.

SNACK:

BASIC MIXED GREENS SALAD

- 1 CUP SHREDDED ROMAINE LETTUCE
- ½ CUP MIXED BABY GREENS
- ½ CUP SHREDDED GREEN LEAF LETTUCE
- ½ CUP SHREDDED RED LEAF LETTUCE
- ¼ CUP SHREDDED RADICCHIO
- ½ CUP PARSLEY
- ¼ CUP ARUGULA

1. Mix all greens together in a bowl. Top with your favorite dressing and enjoy

TURKEY AND AVOCADO WRAP

- 1/4 FRUIT AVOCADO
- 2 OZ SLICED DELI TURKEY

1. Core and cut avocado.
2. Wrap avocado in turkey and enjoy!

BREAKFAST:

HIGH PROTEIN OMELET	
• 4 LARGE EGG WHITE • 2 LARGE EGG • 2 TSP SALT • 2 TSP PEPPER • 3 TBSP BARBECUE SAUCE	1. Whisk eggs, add salt and pepper to taste. 2. Heat a pan with non-stick spray over medium heat. Pour eggs onto pan and cook until most of the egg is turning solid. 3. Fold it in half in pan and let sit for 30 seconds to let inside finish cooking. 4. Add barbecue sauce to taste, enjoy!
BACON	
• 2 STRIPS BACON	1. Cook bacon in a skillet over medium to medium high heat until browned and crisp, turning to brown evenly. 2. Bacon can also be cooked in an oven at 350 degrees for about 20 minutes, or microwave at about 50-60 seconds per strip.
PECANS	
• 1 OZ PECANS	1. Enjoy!

LUNCH:

FLANK STEAK AND TOMATOES	
• 1 DASH CUMIN • 1 DASH SALT • 1 DASH CAYENNE PEPPER • ¼ SPRAY OF COOKING SPRAY • 4 OZ BEEF FLANK • ½ TBSP OLIVE OIL • ¼ TSP OF GARLIC • ¼ JALAPENO PEPPER • .6 OZ TOMATO, CHOPPED • 1 DASH FRESH CILANTRO	1. Preheat broiler to high. 2. In small dish combine half the cumin, half the salt, and cayenne pepper, sprinkle it over the steak. 3. Spray a broiler pan with cooking spray, then place the trimmed flank steak with seasoning in the pan to broil for about 10 minutes, turn once and make sure it is cooked to the proper doneness. Let rest 5 minutes before cutting diagonally across the grain into thin slices. 4. Next, take a large nonstick skillet and heat oil over medium heat. Add the garlic and jalapeno into the pan and allow to cook for 1 minute. Then toss remaining cumin and salt along with the tomatoes into the pan. Allow the tomatoes to soften for 3 minutes, remove them from the heat and stir in cilantro. Serve with steak and enjoy.
TOMATO SOUP	
• ½ CAN TOMATO SOUP • ½ CUP WATER	1. Mix together condensed soup and equal parts water. Microwave 3 minutes and then eat.
FRIED RIPE PLANTAINS	
• 1 MEDIUM PLANTAIN • 1 TBSP VEGETABLE OIL • ½ DASH OF SALT	1. Peel the plantain and cut it diagonally or round, into ¼" slices.

Continued on next page…

2. Drizzle oil into frying pan just enough to coat the bottom of the pan and place on medium heat.
3. When oil begins to shimmer, add plantains, and fry for 1½ minutes on one side, flip and cook for 1 minute on the other side.
4. Remove plantains from pan and rest on paper towels. Sprinkle lightly with salt.

DINNER:

CURRY-STRAWBERRY CHICKEN

- ½ CUP RUSSIAN DRESSING
- ½ TBSP CURRY POWDER
- 1 TSP GRAMS ONION SOUP
- .7 OZ STRAWBERRY JAM
- 4 OZ BONELESS SKINLESS CHICKEN BREAST

1. Mix salad dressing, curry powder, onion soup mix, and strawberry jam in a large bowl until smooth. Place chicken into a baking dish and pour dressing mixture over top. Cover and refrigerate overnight, or at least 1 hour before baking.
2. Preheat oven to 375 degrees.
3. Uncover baking dish. Bake chicken in the preheated oven until no longer pink in center, 2025 minutes.

CELERY

- 2 MEDIUM STALKS CELERY

1. Wash thoroughly and enjoy.

SNACK:

PALEO AVOCADO TUNA SALAD

- 1 FRUIT AVOCADO
- 1 LEMON, YIELDS JUICE
- 1 TBSP CHOPPED ONION
- 5 OZ TUNA
- 1 DASH OF SALT
- 1 DASH OF PEPPER

1. Cut the avocado in half and scoop the middle of each avocado halves into bowl, leaving shell of avocado flesh about ¼ inch thick on each side.
2. Add lemon juice and onion to the avocado in the bowl and mash together. Add drained tuna, salt and pepper to taste, stir to combine.
3. Fill avocado shells with tuna salad to serve.

BANANA

- 1 MEDIUM BANANA

1. Enjoy!

BREAKFAST:

SPINACH AND PEAR OMELET

- 1 TBSP COCONUT OIL
- ½ CUP SPINACH
- 3 LARGE EGGS
- 1 MEDIUM PEAR

1. Lightly grease frying pan with coconut oil and place over medium heat. Add spinach to pan, and cook until wilted, 2-3 minutes.
2. Whisk eggs and pour into pan over spinach. Add
3. pears to the pan and mix everything together well. Cook until eggs whiten, then flip. Cook until

eggs reach desired doneness.

BACON

- 2 STRIPS BACON

1. Cook bacon in a skillet over medium to medium high heat until browned and crisp, turning to brown evenly.

2. Bacon can also be cooked in an oven at 350 degrees for about 20 minutes, or microwave at about 50-60 seconds per strip.

GRILLED PEACHES WITH HONEY

- ½ MEDIUM PEACH
- ½ TSP GRAMS OLIVE OIL
- 1 TSP HONEY

1. Preheat grill to high.
2. Cut peaches in half, remove pits.
3. Brush cut side of peach halves with olive oil and place on grill, cut side down.
4. Grill until golden brown and caramelized, 2-3 minutes.
5. Turn peach halves over and grill until slightly soft and just warmed through, about 2 minutes longer. Remove from grill and drizzle with honey.

LUNCH:

MUSTARD AND SHALLOT SALMON

- ½ TBSP GROUND PEPPER
- ½ TSP SALT
- 1 TBSP MUSTARD SEED
- 8 OZ ATLANTIC SALMON
- ½ TBSP OLIVE OIL

1. Mix the pepper, salt and mustard seed, sprinkle on both sides of fish.
2. Caramelize the shallots in the olive oil on medium heat, about 10-12 minutes. Remove the shallots from heat. Add the salmon. Cook on one side until lightly browned, about 5-7 minutes.
3. Once browned, add ¼ cup water and immediately put on lid. This will steam the fish. Steam for 5-7 minutes and serve.

- 2 ½ SHALLOT

Continued on next page...

ROASTED CHERRY TOMATOES WITH MINT

- 1 TBSP SPEARMINT
- 1 DASH OF SALT
- 1 DASH OF PEPPER
- ½ TBSP OLIVE OIL
- 1 CUP ORGANIC CHERRY TOMATOES

1. Finely chop mint.
2. Preheat oven to 425 degrees.
3. Toss tomatoes with salt, oil, and pepper in a small baking pan and roast in middle of oven until skins just begin to split, 5-10 minutes.
4. Sprinkle tomatoes with mint, enjoy.

DINNER:

CILANTRO LIME SHRIMP

- 1 DASH SALT
- 1 SERRANO PEPPER
- ¼ FRESH CILANTRO
- 2 TBSP LIME JUICE
- 2 TBSP VEGETABLE OIL
- 16 OZ SHRIMP
- 2 GARLIC CLOVES

1. Place a large sauté pan or wok over your strongest burner on high heat. Let pan heat for minute, then add oil. Use a high smoke point oil since you will be cooking the shrimp on very high heat. Let the oil heat until shimmering.
2. Add the chilies to the pan and toss to coat with oil. Cook 30 seconds. Add shrimp and garlic to the pan and sprinkle with salt. Toss to coat with oil. Let the shrimp cook undisturbed for 1 minute before tossing again. Stir-fry until cooked through, about 2-3 minutes.
3. Turn off heat and mix in the cilantro, then the lime juice.
4. Serve hot or at room temperature.

LEMON STEAMED BROCCOLI

- 6 OZ BROCCOLI
- ¼ TSP SALT
- ¼ TSP PEPPER
- ¼ TBSP OLIVE OIL
- 1 DROP LEMON JUICE

1. Trim the broccoli into large florets.
2. Place the broccoli in a steaming basket over boiling water, cover and steam for 3 minutes.
3. Remove lid for a moment, then cook, partially covered, until stems are tender-firm, another 8-10 minutes.
4. Remove to a platter, season with salt, pepper, olive oil and lemon juice.

SNACKS:

MANGO FRUIT SMOOTHIE

- 1 MANGO
- 1 CUP PINEAPPLE CHUNKS
- 1 CUP FROZEN BLUEBERRIES
- 1 CUP WATER

1. Combine all ingredients in a blender and pulse until smooth.

CARROTS

- 1 CUP BABY CARROTS

1. Enjoy by themselves, or with a side of hummus.

BREAKFAST:

BASIC SCRAMBLED EGGS • 3 LARGE EGGS • ½ TBSP OLIVE OIL • ½ TBSP CHOPPED CHIVES • ½ TBSP CHOPPED TARRAGON • ½ DASH OF SALT • ½ DASH OF PEPPER	1. Whisk the eggs in a medium bowl until broken up. Season with a pinch of salt and pepper and beat well. Place 2 tbsp. of the eggs in a small bowl; set aside. 2. Heat a 10-inch nonstick frying pan over medium-low heat until hot, about 2 minutes. Add the butter to the pan and swirl until melted. Pour in larger portion of the eggs, sprinkle with chives and tarragon. Let sit undisturbed until eggs just start to set around edges, about 1-2 minutes. 3. Using rubber spatula, push the eggs from the edges into the center. Let sit again for about 30 seconds, repeat pushing eggs from edges to center every 30 seconds until just set, for a total cooking time of about 5 minutes. 4. Add remaining 2 tbsp. of raw egg until eggs no longer look wet. Remove from heat and season with salt and pepper as needed. Serve immediately.
PALEO BACON WRAPPED PEARS • 1 LARGE PEAR • 4 STRIPS BACON	1. Preheat oven to 400 degrees. Cover a large rimmed baking sheet with aluminum foil. Leaving skin on, cut each pear into quarters. 2. Wrap each quarter of pear with a slice of bacon and place on baking sheet. Bake for 25 3. minutes, or until bacon is crispy.
APPLE • 1 MEDIUM APPLE	2. Simply wash and enjoy.

Continued on next page…

SIMPLE CARROT SOUP

- ½ TBSP COCONUT OIL
- ¼ MEDIUM ONION
- 1 TSP CURRY PASTE
- 8 OZ CHOPPED CARROTS
- ½ CUP COCONUT MILK
- ¼ TSP SALT
- 3 OZ WATER
- ¼ LEMON
- 1 DASH FRESH CILANTRO
- .4 OZ ALMONDS

1. In a large soup pan over medium-high heat add the coconut oil and onion.
2. Stir until onions are well-coated, and allow to sauté until translucent, a few minutes. Stir in the curry paste, and then the carrots. Allow to cook another minute or two, and then add the coconut milk, salt, and water, adding more water to cover if needed.
3. Allow to simmer until the carrots are tender, 10-15 minutes, and then puree using a blender, until soup is completely smooth.
4. This next part is important with any soup. Make any needed adjustments. Add more water if the consistency needs to be thinned out a bit. After that taste for salt, adding more if needed.
5. Season with a squeeze of lemon juice. Serve garnished with cilantro and almonds. Enjoy.

DINNER:

EASY GRILLED CHICKEN TERIYAKI

- 8 OZ BONELESS SKINLESS CHICKEN BREASTS
- ½ CUP TERIYAKI SAUCE
- 2 TBSP LEMON JUICE
- 1 TSP GARLIC
- 1 TSP SESAME OIL

1. Place chicken, teriyaki sauce, lemon juice, garlic, and sesame oil in a large resealable plastic bag. Seal bag and shake to coat. Place
2. in refrigerator for 24 hours, turning every so often.
   Preheat grill to high heat.
3. Lightly oil the grill grate. Remove chicken from bag, discarding any remaining marinade. Grill for 6-8 minutes on each side, or until juices run clear when chicken is pierced with a fork.

BAKED AND DRESSED ZUCCHINI

- 2 SMALL ZUCCHINIS
- 1 TSP OLIVE OIL
- 1 DASH SALT
- 1 DASH PEPPER
- ½ TBSP RED WINE VINEGAR
- 1 DROP PEPPERMINT

1. Preheat oven to 400 degrees.
2. Give the zucchini a good wash and pat dry. In a baking dish, toss the zucchinis with the olive oil and a generous dash of salt and pepper.
3. Bake the zucchini for 15 minutes until soft and skin has blistered.
4. Once out of the oven, dress with a couple o splashes of red wine vinegar and the chopped mint. Add more olive oil and salt and pepper if desired.

SNACK:

GREEN GODDESS JUICE

- 1 MEDIUM APPLE
- 1 MEDIUM CUCUMBER
- ½ HEAD LETTUCE
- 4 CUPS CHOPPED KALE
- 1 ½ CUP SPINACH
- 2 ½ MEDIUM STALK CELERY
- ½ LEMON
- 1 TBSP COCONUT WATER
- 1 DASH STEVIA SWEETENER

1. Juice all the fruits and vegetables.
2. Add coconut water and stevia to taste and mix.

CAULIFLOWER AND TAHINI

- 1 CUP CHOPPED CAULIFLOWER
- 2 TBSP SESAME TAHINI

1. Chop the cauliflower lovingly, to retain some of the florets.
2. Serve the cauliflower pieces with tahini for dipping. Enjoy!

BREAKFAST:

COCONUT FLOUR PANCAKES

- 1 MEDIUM BANANA
- 1 LARGE EGG
- 2 TBSP EGG WHITE
- ¼ TSP BAKING SODA
- 1 TSP VINEGAR
- ½ TSP VANILLA EXTRACT
- 2 TSP COCONUT FLOUR
- 1 SPRAY PAM COOKING SPRAY

1. Heat skillet to medium-high heat. Mash bananas in a liquid measuring cup with pour spout. Add in eggs and whisk until well combined.
2. Stir in baking soda/vinegar and vanilla if desired. Stir in coconut flour.
3. Lightly grease skillet. Pour pancake sized amount of batter into skillet. Allow to cook on one side until fluffy and bubbly in center. Flip and cook on other side until evenly browned.

LUNCH:

EGG SALAD

- 4 LARGE EGGS
- ¼ LIGHT MAYONNAISE
- ½ TSP PEPPER
- 1 DASH PAPRIKA
- 3 TSP OLIVES

1. Place eggs in a medium saucepan with enough cold water to cover and bring to a boil.
2. Cover the saucepan, remove from heat, and let eggs stand in hot water for 10-12 minutes. Remove from hot water, cool, peel, and chop.
3. In a large bowl, mix eggs, mayo, pepper, and paprika. Mash with a potato masher or fork until smooth. Gently stir in the olives. Refrigerate until serving.

GRILLED POLENTA CHIPS

- 4 OZ. YELLOW POLENTA
- ½ TBSP OLIVE OIL
- 1 TBSP NUTRITIONAL YEAST
- ½ DASH OF PEPPER
- ½ DASH OF SALT

1. Heat a grill pan to medium-high heat and lightly rub your grill with olive oil.
2. Cut tube of polenta into ¼ to ½ inch slices. Brush both sides of the polenta cakes with the olive oil.
3. Sprinkle both sides with nutritional yeast, salt, and pepper.

Continued on next page…

4. Lay the polenta rounds in one layer on the grill, and grill for 5 minutes on each side or until both sides are golden and crunchy and have grill marks.

5. Remove the cakes from the grill and place on a large plate to cool. Serve warm or at room temperature.

DINNER:

AVOCADO STUFFED BURGERS
- 5 OZ GROUND BEEF
- 1/3 FRUIT AVOCADO
- .3 OZ SUN DRIED TOMATOES
- 1 TSP LEMON JUICE
- 1 DROP LEMON ZEST
- 1 DASH OF PEPPER
- 1 DASH OF SALT

1. Preheat grill to medium-medium high heat.

2. Put ground beef in a large mixing bowl and add black pepper, 1 teaspoon salt, and the zest of one lemon. Mix well. Using your hands, form into thin patties. Make sure to make an even number of patties.

3. In separate bowl combine avocados, chopped sun dried tomatoes, lemon juice, and salt. Mash the avocados and mix ingredients well to get as smooth as you prefer.

4. Place your avocado mixture on top of the bottom of half of the burger, ensuring you leave room to seal the burgers without it leaking out.

5. Place top patties over the top of your mixture and pinch the edges of burgers all the way around to seal.

6. Grill burgers to your liking, about 6-8 minutes per side. Ensure you cook evenly on both sides. When done grilling, allow your burger to rest for 10 minutes and then serve.

Continued on next page…

TOMATO SOUP
- ½ CAN TOMATO SOUP
- ½ CUP WATER

1. Mix together soup and equal parts water. Microwave for 3 minutes and then enjoy.

ZUCCHINI SPEARS
- 1 DASH SALT
- 1 ZUCCHINI

1. Cut zucchini lengthwise and cut into ¼ inch wedges.
2. Cook zucchini in boiled and salted water until crisp tender, about 1 minute. Drain and sprinkle with salt.

SNACK:

LIME CHICKEN SALAD
- 5 OZ CANNED CHICKEN
- 2 TSP LIME JUICE
- 1 DASH OF SALT
- 4 LARGE LETTUCE LEAVES

1. Combine the chicken, lime juice, and salt.
2. Arrange the bib leaves and serve the chicken salad on top. Enjoy!

CAULIFLOWER AND TAHINI
- 1 CUP CHOPPED CAULIFLOWER
- 2 TBSP SESAME TAHINI

1. Chop the cauliflower lovingly, to retain some of the florets.
2. Serve the cauliflower pieces with tahini for dipping. Enjoy!

<u>Note:</u> Above is one full day "substitute" meal plan that can be used to interchange any day in Restore week (Tuesday through Friday). Choose this substitute meal plan if you want and substitute it in for any day you choose.

BREAKFAST:

COCONUT FLOUR PANCAKES
- 1 MEDIUM BANANA
- 1 LARGE EGG
- 2 TBSP EGG WHITE
- ¼ TSP BAKING SODA
- 1 TSP VINEGAR
- ½ TSP VANILLA EXTRACT
- 2 TSP COCONUT FLOUR
- 1 SPRAY PAM COOKING SPRAY

1. Heat skillet to medium-high heat. Mash bananas in a liquid measuring cup with pour spout. Add in eggs and whisk until well combined.
2. Stir in baking soda/vinegar and vanilla if desired. Stir in coconut flour.
3. Lightly grease skillet. Pour pancake sized amount of batter into skillet. Allow to cook on one side until fluffy and bubbly in center. Flip and cook on other side until evenly browned.

LUNCH:

EGG SALAD
- 4 LARGE EGGS
- ¼ LIGHT MAYONNAISE
- ½ TSP PEPPER
- 1 DASH PAPRIKA
- .5 OZ OLIVES

1. Place eggs in a medium saucepan with enough cold water to cover and bring to a boil.
2. Cover the saucepan, remove from heat, and let eggs stand in hot water for 10-12 minutes. Remove from hot water, cool, peel, and chop.
3. In a large bowl, mix eggs, mayo, pepper, and paprika. Mash with a potato masher or fork until smooth. Gently stir in the olives.
4. Refrigerate until serving.

GRILLED POLENTA CHIPS
- 4 OZ YELLOW POLENTA
- ½ TBSP OLIVE OIL
- 1 TBSP NUTRITIONAL YEAST
- ½ DASH OF PEPPER
- ½ DASH OF SALT

1. Heat a grill pan to medium-high heat and lightly rub your grill with olive oil.
2. Cut tube of polenta into ¼ to ½ inch slices. Brush both sides of the polenta cakes with the olive oil. Sprinkle both sides with nutritional yeast, salt, and pepper.
3. Lay the polenta rounds in one layer on the grill, and grill for 5 minutes on each side or until both sides are golden and crunchy and have grill marks.
4. Remove the cakes from the grill and place on a large plate to cool. Serve warm or at room temperature.

Continued on next page…

DINNER:

AVOCADO STUFFED BURGERS

- 5 OZ GROUND BEEF
- 1/3 FRUIT AVOCADO
- .3 OZ SUN DRIED TOMATOES
- 1 TSP LEMON JUICE
- 1 DROP LEMON ZEST
- 1 DASH OF PEPPER
- 1 DASH OF SALT

1. Preheat grill to medium-medium high heat. Put ground beef in a large mixing bowl and add black pepper, 1 teaspoon salt, and the zest of one lemon. Mix well. Using your hands, form into thin patties.
2. Make sure to make an even number of patties. In separate bowl combine avocados, chopped sun dried tomatoes, lemon juice, and salt. Mash the avocados and mix ingredients well to get as smooth as you prefer.
3. Place your avocado mixture on top of the bottom of half of the burger, ensuring you leave room to seal the burgers without it leaking out.
4. Place top patties over the top of your mixture and pinch the edges of burgers all the way around to seal.
5. Grill burgers to your liking, about 6-8 minutes per side. Ensure you cook evenly on both sides. When done grilling, allow your burger to rest for 10 minutes and then serve.

TOMATO SOUP

- ½ CAN TOMATO SOUP
- ½ CUP WATER

1. Mix together soup and equal parts water. Microwave for 3 minutes and then enjoy.

ZUCCHINI SPEARS

- 1 DASH SALT
- 1 ZUCCHINI

1. Cut zucchini lengthwise and cut into ¼ inch wedges.
2. Cook zucchini in boiled and salted water until crisp tender, about 1 minute. Drain and sprinkle with salt.

SNACK:

LIME CHICKEN SALAD

- 1 CAN CHICKEN
- 2 TSP LIME JUICE
- 1 DASH OF SALT
- 4 LARGE LETTUCE LEAVES

1. Combine the chicken, lime juice, and salt.
2. Arrange the bib leaves and serve the chicken salad on top.

CAULIFLOWER AND TAHINI

- 1 CUP CHOPPED CAULIFLOWER
- 2 TBSP SESAME TAHINI

1. Chop the cauliflower lovingly, to retain some of the florets.
2. Serve the cauliflower pieces with tahini for dipping.

Note: Above is one full day "substitute" meal plan that can be used to interchange any day in Restore week (Tuesday through Friday). Choose this substitute meal plan if you want and substitute it in for any day you choose.

FOOD ITEM	AVERAGE SERVING SIZE	CALORIES
PROTEIN		
HAMBURGER PATTY	3.5 OZ	235 CAL
TRI TIP	3.5 OZ	182 CAL
PORK CUTLET	3.5 OZ	231 CAL
CHICKEN	4 OZ	190 CAL
BEEF NEW YORK STRIP STEAK	4 OZ	220 CAL
BABY BACK RIBS	3 OZ	270 CAL
PORK SIRLOIN	3 OZ	168 CAL
BEEF RIBEYE STEAK	6 OZ	450 CAL
SALMON	3 OZ	200 CAL
HALIBUT	3 OZ	107 CAL
FRIED EGG	1 LARGE EGG	92 CAL
BOILED EGG	1 LARGE EGG	77 CAL
SCRAMBLED EGG	1 LARGE EGG	101 CAL
CARBOHYDRATES		
BANANA	1 MEDIUM BANANA	104 CAL
APPLE	1 MEDIUM APPLE	80 CAL
ORANGE	1 FRUIT	69 CAL
SPAGHETTI WITH MEAT SAUCE	10 OZ	286 CAL
CHICKEN ALFREDO PASTA	8.14 OZ	321 CAL
WHITE RICE	1 CUP	205 CAL
BROWN RICE	1 CUP	216 CAL
BLACK BEANS	½ CUP	90 CAL
REFRIED BEANS	½ CUP	125 CAL
PINTO BEANS	½ CUP	144 CAL
BROCCOLI	1 CUP	65 CAL
GREEN BEANS	1 CUP	25 CAL
CORN	4 OZ	153 CAL
WHOLE WHEAT BREAD	1 SLICE	69 CAL
WHITE BREAD	1 SLICE	120 CAL
SOURDOUGH BREAD	1 SLICE	120 CAL
RESTAURANTS		
IN N OUT BURGER WITH ONION	1 SERVING	390 CAL

MCDONALDS CHEESEBURGER	1 SERVING	300 CAL
TACO BELL CRUNCHY SUPREME TACO	1 SERVING	190 CAL
TACO BELL BEAN BURRITO	1 SERVING	370 CAL
EL POLLO LOCO AL CARBON CHICKEN TACOS	1 SERVING	160 CAL
JAMBA JUICE ACAI PRIMO FRUIT BOWL	1 SERVING	540 CAL
CARL'S JR SPICY CHICKEN SANDWICH	1 SERVING	460 CAL
SUBWAY HAM SANDWICH 6 INCH	1 SERVING	450 CAL
PANERA BREAD STRAWBERRY POPPYSEED CHICKEN SALAD	1 SERVING	350 CAL
RED LOBSTER STARTER SAMPLER	1 SERVING	620 CAL
OLIVE GARDEN CHICKEN ALFREDO FETTUCCINE	1 SERVING	500 CAL
RED ROBIN WINGS	1 SERVING	1,023 CAL
APPLEBEE'S TRIPLE BACON BURGER	1 SERVING	1,190 CAL

Note: Above is an example of some but not all food items allowed in Combo.
Remember you can eat anything you want in Combo (Saturday and Sunday) as
long as you stay within your targeted caloric intake.

RECIPE: COMBO   *SATURDAY- SUNDAY: 2,500 CALORIES*

SATURDAY BREAKFAST:

- 2 CHOCOLATE DONUTS
  (740 CALORIES)
- CARAMEL MACCHIATO COFFEE,
  STARBUCKS
  (190 CALORIES)

SATURDAY LUNCH:

- 1 JIMMY JOHN BLT
  (441 CALORIES)
- 1 BAKED LAYS CHIP SNACK BAG
  (100 CALORIES)
- 8 FL OZ SODA
  (119 CALORIES)

SATURDAY DINNER:

- 1 SERVING PASTA FETTUCCINE ALFREDO,
  OLIVE GARDEN
  (500 CALORIES)
- 2 BREAD STICKS, OLIVE GARDEN
  (300 CALORIES)
- 8 FL OZ PINK LEMONADE
  (100 CALORIES)

TOTAL: 2,490 CALORIES

SUNDAY BREAKFAST:

- 1 SERVING BREAKFAST BURRITO
  (700 CALORIES)

SUNDAY LUNCH:

- 6 TACOS AL CARBON, EL POLLO LOCO
  (960 CALORIES)

SUNDAY DINNER:

- 3 CUPS CHICKEN AND VEGGIE STIR FRY
  (690 CALORIES)
- 1 BEER
  (153 CALORIES)

TOTAL: 2,503 CALORIES

<u>Note</u>: In Combo you can eat ANY food, but stay in your caloric intake!

Testimonials

"The best thing about the Macro Circuit Diet is the recipe meal plan or quick start meal plan. This was very handy for me because on those busy days I followed the quick start plan, but when I had time, I switched to a recipe meal plan which kept things exciting for me. Very lifestyle friendly!"

-Cara Hix

"I'm now so happy with my results after switching from my own "not knowing what to do" plan which was completely frustrating, to my awesome Macro Circuit Diet. This diet is so user and lifestyle friendly, it makes my nutrition program fun, plus I'm making all kinds of results. I finally found something that works and that I can stay on. I highly recommend MCD."

-Dianna Gunn

"The expertise that comes from Leo through the Macro Circuit Diet is incredible. His knowledge about nutrition is so encouraging which gives me the confidence knowing that reaching my health and fitness goals will be attainable. I'm so blessed to have found the Macro Circuit Diet."

-Ambrea Flores

"Macro Circuit Diet is such an easy program to follow. Can't wait to see more transformation in the upcoming months!"

-Martina Van Der Vorst

"I've been on the Macro Circuit Diet coming up on a year and can really see the difference. So glad I made the commitment to start this plan."

-Lisa Vieira

"At the end of 2016, I was at a really low place in my life. I was severely overweight and generally unhappy. I decided I wanted to take control of my life and in Jan. 2017 I began the Macro Circuit Diet. This diet is amazing and very user friendly. So far, I've been following this program for 3 months and have lost 25 lbs and even more inches. While I'm still overweight, I'm now confident I will reach my health and fitness goals as long as I have MCD. Highly recommend it!"

–Lariane Castro

Dehydration and inflammation kill your immune system

Your body is built to be resilient, yet most are unaware of the triggers which are mostly self- inflicted slowly breaking the body down. When these triggers become chronic, the mind and body become overwhelmed. In this state the physiology can become dehydrated and inflamed creating an environment that creates havoc on the immune system. This condition exposes the physiology to the fight or flight response where it perceives a threat. In this state, your body will alert you, however most individuals are unaware, or ignore these signals which can expose them to great harm. Things that cause dehydration and inflammation are extreme behavior. A lifestyle change is of most importance. Weaponize your immune system with herbs.

In order to make your immune system as strong as possible, creating that extra shield, adding herbs to your nutritional regimen is vital. Herbs have antiviral properties which are a major player for fighting off viral infections, in addition effective against a wide range of viruses. Foods that fit this criteria include garlic, olive leaf, ginger, oregano, spirulina, Shiitake mushrooms, green tea, elderberries, yogurt.

Full Body Thru Space/ Resistance Training

The body is designed to move, or it dies. Walking is one of the best things you can do to move your body thru space which mitigates muscle loss, improves muscle endurance and tone, and strengthens vital organs. But if you want to strengthen your immune system to even a higher level, implementing a resistance exercise regimen using your body thru space will add an extra shield of defense for your immune system. It takes a commitment of three hours per week, training bands, ball, stick, dumbbells ranging from 5-25, which are optional.

Part 3

Automatic Body Balance Training

Automatic Body Balance Training System is an interesting and exciting new product which has been designed as a result of form following function. It's always been known that athletes who have better balance are better performing athletes, which is why throughout a sports specific training program, athletes perform exercises requiring balance for proper execution.

Guaranteed Fitness Plus has taken unique qualities of a sports specific training program and developed Automatic Body Balance Training System to target those individuals who are not necessarily interested in

188

becoming high-level performing athletes; however, are interested in developing strength, better balance, and better body awareness. I developed this program with first hand knowledge. I have been an athlete all my life and have found it extremely encouraging even now in my 50's, that I'm still able to compete and have the *energy* to keep up with athletes much younger.

The reason for this success is that I've kept to a regular exercise and nutrition routine. What has been even a bigger surprise is how healthy I am, how good I feel and that compared to people of my own age I generally look younger. It's a well known fact that regular physical activity slows down the aging process. In addition, it's also a fact that exercise doesn't need to be strenuous, but it does need to be consistent.

Regular exercise is the fountain of youth because it either reduces, decreases or combats things that shorten our lifespan such as arthritis, heart disease, depression, anxiety, stress, and blood pressure, just to name a few. It improves restorative sleep, mind function and increases the immune system. There is no down side. It's important for people to understand that they have a good degree of control over the future of their body despite genetics.

The MacArthur Foundation Study revealed in some interesting research that habits are more important than heredity. This is really good news considering that too many people use what they think are bad genes as an excuse for their poor health.

It _is_ possible to be vibrant and healthy as we get older.

I've seen this first hand and I'm counting on it. I'm not afraid of getting older; in fact, I'm looking forward to it with a positive attitude.I have developed The Automatic Body Balance Training System for this very reason. This program is specifically designed for the more mature adult. Automatic Body Balance Training System is very versatile. For example, you don't necessarily need any fancy gym equipment; in fact, it can be done in the comfort of your own home or your favorite local gym.

A very specific and complete training routine has been developed using only your body as the source of resistance, which is extremely efficient, if proper angles and certain body positions are implemented.

There are also specific training routines in the Automatic Body Balance Training System that can be used with equipment such as light dumbbells, rubber bands, and stability balls. Every one of the routines, with or without equipment, is extremely effective. In a short time, individuals using this unique training system will develop better strength, balance, and better body awareness. The risk of injury will be reduced and confidence will be increased. Automatic Body Balance Training System also benefits those who are interested in building endurance, strength, and minimizing the effects of osteoporosis. Too many times, people fall because of poor balance and brittle bones.

One may not want to run a marathon; however, one does want to enjoy life's hard-earned rewards. To pick up a grandchild, to enjoy a vacation or to stroll along the beach should all be pleasurable activities to look forward to, not dreaded or worse yet not even contemplated.

With minimal effort, the body can maintain muscle, strength and flexibility. <u>Prevention</u> and <u>maintenance</u> make it so the body can continue to function for a healthy and active lifestyle.

Leo

The Product

Micro Circuit Training™ is a life transforming technology that will impact individuals by changing how they look and feel, quickly and automatically. This is how the product name (Automatic Body Balance Training) evolved. Automatic Body Balance Training is so efficient, an individual can achieve maximum fitness in as little as three hours per week.

Automatic Body Balance is unique, because it takes the critical elements which are responsible for changing the body, and it implements a complete exercise and nutrition strategy.

This means setting up a complete exercise and nutrition program that takes advantage of all the training elements that change the body in the most efficient way. The primary training components (known as the three training areas) are resistance training, cardio conditioning, and nutrition.

However, Automatic Body Balance Training System takes the three training areas to another level. It is important to include specific training phases into each training area. At certain times in an exercise program, the training should accelerate to diminish potential plateaus. It's important to have an exercise program that has structure, without killing the variety and creativity that is necessary for the continuation of an ongoing program that will always produce results.

Automatic Body Balance Training considers all of the training variables and is specific. It is a complete training system that can be used by anyone who wants to quickly improve the body's level of fitness. Automatic Body Balance Training takes absolutely all of the guess-work out of every part of a training program, and this allows the individuals to know without question that they are on the right training program.

One major reason for this is that there are well-established principles of adaptation, and the body will always respond if the right kind of training and nutrition stimuli is applied.

The way Automatic Body Balance Training is designed, it is virtually impossible for the body to ever hit plateaus where flexibility, balance, and strength gains are stopped. Automatic Body Balance is an exercise and nutrition program that will change its stimuli automatically throughout a workout program based upon the individual's level in his or her fitness program.

**Easy, Simple, and Flexible
 Implementation**

 Automatic Body Balance Training is easy to implement and is very flexible. It typically involves three workouts per week: Monday, Wednesday, and Friday. One can work out on any three days. However, if one would like to train three days in a row, or two days in a row with a day's rest in between that is fine. The training session lasts one hour: 30 minutes of weight training and 30 minutes of cardio.

It doesn't matter which is performed first. Cardio can be done in the beginning as a warm-up, for five minutes or even for 15 minutes, with the balance of the cardio session

being completed after the weight training
session. It's easy, simple, and flexible.
and Finally..

The information, knowledge and results
individuals will receive and gain from
Automatic Body Balance Training and the
invention of MCT™ will be powerful and life
changing. The techniques, training philosophy
and design of this unique system have been
tried and tested on thousands of clients and
always work and produce results.

Equipment List

	Adjustable Flat Bench
	Dumbbells ranging from 2-20 lbs.
	Platform
	Stability Ball
	Ankle Weights 1.5-3.0 lbs.
	Rubber Bands
	Body Bar
	Medicine Ball ranging from 8-11 lbs
	Workout Stick
	Chair
	Heart Rate Monitor
	Chin Up Bar

Above is a list of equipment needed to perform all of the exercises in the Automatic Body Balance Training System.

The Invention of
Micro Circuit Training™

Micro Circuit Training (MCT) ™ is a unique technology in exercise and nutrition which emphasizes three elements known as the three training areas: resistance training, cardiovascular conditioning, and nutrition
All of the guess-work has been taken out of what kind of exercise, cardio, and nutritional program that should be followed.

The Three Training Areas

There are three training areas in the exercise program, all of which are critical for achieving maximum fitness.

-Resistance Training

-Cardiovascular Conditioning

-Nutrition

All three training areas are necessary. Leaving even <u>one</u> of these areas out of an exercise program will compromise overall results.

The primary functions of resistance training are to tone or build muscle as well as improve metabolic functioning along with enhancing the body's ability for quicker recovery from workouts.

The primary functions of cardiovascular conditioning are to burn fat, and to eliminate the lactic acid created from weight-training sessions; this helps speed up recovery for upcoming workouts.

The primary functions of nutrition are energy sourcing the body with adequate fuel for high-energy workouts, keeping it healthy, and helping the body recover from workouts, not to mention, its function for promoting fat loss and muscle gain.

Micro Circuit Resistance Training™

 Micro Circuit Training™ is a 20-30 minute workout, which experience has shown to be the optimum period for it. The strategy behind MCT™ is to train multiple body parts together.

One will discover that MCT™ is a very effective and efficient way to do a lot of work in a short period of time. It is designed to be an up tempo workout program, which keeps an individual moving. Body parts are grouped in a circuit in such a way for the individual to do a lot of exercise without having to spend very much time resting.

Generally MCT™ consists of three circuits. <u>Three different exercises are done in each circuit</u>. The same body part may be trained in the circuit, providing that different exercises are being performed. <u>Each time a circuit is performed this is defined as a training round</u>. <u>There are three training rounds in each training session</u>.

Repetitions may range from 8-15. It all depends upon the particular week the individual is working on.

The sequence of exercises in each circuit can be modified at any moment, which is helpful when working in busy health clubs.

Because of the flexibility of MCT™, there never is a problem with an individual not getting a great workout or with the training tempo getting interrupted or bogged down by other people working out in a crowded gym.

Micro Circuit Training™ is designed to be a very efficient resistance training program.

In order for the body to change, it must be challenged, without being overwhelmed. MCT™ does this because the client utilizing this training methodology is doing a lot of work in each one of the training circuits.

The body parts trained within each circuit are sequenced in a way that fatigues the muscle being trained thoroughly while allowing recovery for the other body parts that are a part of the training circuit.

The other advantage of MCT™ is that rest periods are kept to a minimum. A 20-30 minute MCT™ session can be used by individuals who are novices or highly trained athletes.

The way that a circuit should be executed is that the first exercise is performed for a certain amount of repetitions and then one immediately moves to the second exercise, performing the repetitions designated, then moving on to the third exercise. After the third exercise is completed in the circuit, a rest period of approximately 30-45 seconds or can vary according to the individual's ability to recover.

In each micro circuit, the repetitions can be the same or completely different for each body part. MCT™ is designed to be extremely flexible and efficient. The most important thing an individual should always emphasize when resistance training is that the body part being trained is thoroughly fatigued, but not overworked.

MCT™ Cardio Training

Cardiovascular training is the second component of the three training areas that are part of the Micro Circuit Training™ system. MCT™ cardiovascular training has five training phases over a 12 week training program that specifically corresponds with micro circuit resistance training.

The MCT™ cardiovascular training phases are executed in a specific order to develop the full potential of the individual, in order to maximize fitness results. It is important to understand that the body is always trying to adapt to its environment. So MCT™ cardio is constantly being manipulated in order to keep the body off guard which produces terrific and consistent results.

The Best Cardio Exercise?

There really isn't one cardio exercise that is more effective than another. Some individuals will have a personal preference, and some will have a more difficult time with a certain cardio exercise because of a pre-existing injury. Otherwise, in terms of body fat loss, all cardio is pretty equal. There is high-and low-impact cardio. Running and/ or high- intensity aerobic classes are two high impact activities which can be hard on the body's joints, ligaments, and tendons. Some individuals can tolerate high-impact cardio, while others cannot.

Stationary bikes, elliptical machines, and walking are examples of low-impact cardio. Both high-and low-impact cardio are effective. The top four cardio exercise machines that can be used in most gyms or health clubs are treadmills, stationary bikes, Stairmaster equipment, and elliptical machines. If there is no cardio equipment available, it is always possible to walk or run outdoors. It is recommended that if an individual is predisposed to or has joint problems, he or she do low-impact cardio or walk or run on a padded track.

Cardiovascular Conditioning Defined

The body utilizes two different energy systems, one aerobic and the other anaerobic. By definition, aerobic means with oxygen and anaerobic means without oxygen.

The real difference between anaerobic and aerobic conditioning is how the body utilizes energy. The body primarily uses fat as its energy source when in an <u>aerobic state.</u> When the body is in an <u>anaerobic state</u>, it utilizes glucose as its primary energy source Individuals must understand the importance of the two different energy systems and how they should be applied properly to their training program.

When doing aerobic activity the heart rate must be in a training target zone ranging between 70%-85% of an individual's maximum heart rate. The reason for the aerobic training target zone is to ensure that the body does not cross over into an anaerobic state of conditioning.

If this should happen during an aerobic activity, then the body will now begin to utilize glucose as its energy, rather than fat, which defeats the main purpose.

It is a common mistake for individuals to do cardio while utilizing the wrong energy system, meaning that they are in an <u>anaerobic</u> state of conditioning, rather than <u>aerobic.</u>

This happens mistakenly because individuals think that when doing cardio, working harder is better, because that will burn more body fat. Working hard is fine; however, the heart rate must be in the training target zone to be most efficient in utilizing fat burning for energy.

The maximum heart rate of an individual is age dependent, which means that aerobic training target zones vary according to age. A simple formula listed below will ensure that the proper heart rate is being maintained.

Note
The rule of thumb is that aerobic training target zones range between 70%-85% of an individual's maximum heart rate. This is recommended; however, it is important to understand that as an individual is getting in better cardiovascular condition, the aerobic training target zone can expand.

The Aerobic Heart Rate Formula

The formula below shows how to arrive at an ideal heart range for burning body fat:

Step (1)   220 minus age equals maximum heart rate.

Step (2)   Max heart rate times 0.7 equals low end ideal heart rate to burn body fat.

Step (3)   Max heart rate times 0.85 yields the high end ideal heart rate to burn body fat.

Cardio Schedule

Cardiovascular conditioning is the second component of the three training areas of MCT™. It is important to execute and implement cardio throughout MCT™. Below is a cardio schedule that is designed to coordinate with MCT™ resistance training.

Weeks 1 & 2 -In the first two weeks, cardio is done for 15 minutes before the resistance-training session and for another 15 minutes afterwards. It should be done three days per week. Heart rate should be kept between 65% - 70% of one's maximum.

Weeks 3 & 4 - Cardio is done for 30 minutes all at one time. It can be done before or after the resistance training session. Cardio is done three days per week. Heart rate should be kept between 75% - 80% of one's maximum.

Weeks 5 & 6 - Cardio intensity is increased because the heart rate is at a higher target range. Cardio is done for 30 minutes all at one time, either before or after the resistance training, and performed three days per week. Heart rate should be kept between 80% - 85% of one's maximum.

Week 7 - Cardio intensity is reduced because the heart rate is at a lower target range. It should be performed three days per week for 30 minutes each time all at one time, either before or after resistance training. Heart rate should be between 65% - 70% of one's maximum.

Weeks 8 & 9 - Cardio for weeks 8 & 9 will be interval training. During Week 8, cardio will be done four days per week for 30 minutes, and intervals will be done every five minutes. In the

first five minutes, cardio will be increased so the heart rate is at 85% of one's maximum.
 During the next 10 minutes, cardio is reduced, so the heart rate is at 65% -70% of maximum. In Week 9, there will be two 10- minute intervals with a five minute recovery. During the 10- minute ramping interval, heart rate will be at 85% of maximum. During the five minute recovery period, heart rate will be at 65% - 70% of maximum.

Example of Intervals during Weeks 8 & 9

Week 8 - A five minute interval at heart rate (HR) - 85% → Recovery 10 minutes HR 65% - 70% → 5 minute interval HR →85% - Recovery 10 minutes - end of cardio.
Week 9 - A 10-minute interval at heart rate (HR) 85% → Recovery 5 minutes HR 65% - 70% → 10-minute interval HR 85% - Recovery 5 minutes HR 65% - 70% - end workout.
Week 10 - Cardio for week 10 is performed three days per week, for 30 minutes each time. Heart rate will be kept at 65%-70% of maximum.
Week 11 - Cardio is performed three days per week, for 30 minutes each time. Heart rate will be kept at 75%-80% of maximum.
Week 12 - Cardio is performed three days per

week, for 30 minutes each time. Heart rate will be kept at 65%-70% of maximum.

Diet and Nutrition Schedule

Diet and nutrition is one of three elements which must be implemented in a certain order to maximize overall performance. Below is a diet and nutrition schedule, which can be implemented with or without exercise.

There is a tremendous amount of confusion in the diet and nutrition industry, especially when it comes to knowing what type of diet or nutrition program should be followed.

First, it must be understood that our body functions and operates off of two metabolisms. Specifically it's either one or the other:

1. Free Fatty Acid Metabolism
2. Glucose Metabolism

In order to determine which metabolism is dominant, a diet analysis must be performed on the individual by a doctor or dietitian.

If a person is consuming on a daily basis 30 grams of carbohydrates or less, the Free Fatty Acid Metabolism is dominant. If daily carbohydrate consumption is above 30 grams, the Glucose Metabolism is dominant.

The diet analysis will also serve as a tool to determine daily calorie consumption, which will be useful when determining which calorie category the individual should be put.

Both metabolisms are effective and can be incorporated throughout MCT™. But in order to maximize results, only one type of diet should be followed at a time, which should be determined by the individual's physician or dietitian.

Diet and nutrition is the third component of the three training areas which comprise the MCT™ system.

Calorie Categories

MCT™ diet and nutrition has three specific calorie categories: Weight Loss, Weight Maintenance and Weight Gain, which have calorie ranges for males and females, depending on their fitness goal.

These three categories will apply to both male and female, but with some differences. Men, because of their ability to produce testosterone, naturally carry more muscle

mass, which requires more calories to maintain the body. Below is a calorie breakdown in the three categories for men and women:
Week 1 The emphasis should be on getting acclimated to the resistance training and cardio conditioning. Also, during week 1, a two day food journal should be filled out. A diet analysis should be completed by a dietician to determine the nutrition schedule the individual should follow.

Men	Weight Loss (calorie decrease)	1500 - 1800 calories
Men	Weight Maintenance	1800 – 2500calories
Men	Weight Gain (calorie increase)	2500 - 3000 calories
Women	Weight Loss (calorie decrease)	1000 - 1200 calories
Women	Weight Maintenance	1200 - 1500 calories
Women	Weight Gain (calorie increase)	1500 - 2000 calories

Weeks 2 and 3 If the weight goal is to lose,

then a decrease in calories during these two weeks should be implemented, which will put the individual in the weight loss category.

Weeks 4 and 5 During these two weeks, calories will be increased to the weight maintenance category for two weeks.

Weeks 6 and 7 If at this point, the weight goal is not reached; a calorie reduction should be implemented back to the weight loss category.

Weeks 8 and 9 Calories increase back to the weight maintenance category.

 Weeks 10, 11 and 12 If the weight goal has not been reached, calories will be decreased back to the weight loss category. These three weeks will be the most intense in terms of calorie reduction, in part because of the length of time.

Explanation
 There are specific weeks where calorie reductions are implemented in order to stimulate the metabolism for those individuals who need it. If individuals are on schedule, with their weight goals, it is not necessary to implement calorie reductions in the designated weeks. One could stay in the weight

maintenance category throughout the entire
program.

For those individuals who are interested in
gaining weight, then in the specific weeks
designated for a calorie reduction, a calorie
increase would be implemented. In this
scenario, the individual is in the weight gain
category and then returns to weight
maintenance.

The Four Training Components

1. Individual's Fitness Level - There are three levels of
fitness: novice, intermediate, and advanced. This
indicates the level of experience that the individual has
with regard to diet and exercise.

2. Exercise Selection - Choosing the right exercises to
perform throughout your training program makes the
training experience a greatly productive one every
time.

In order for the exercises to produce maximum
results, training circuits have been
predetermined with a wide variety of exercises.
The training circuits are designed to be specific
to the five training phases which range from

the novice to the advanced client.

 3. Exercise Selection - Choosing the right exercises to perform throughout your training program makes the training experience a greatly productive one every time. To help you do the most productive exercises, predetermined training circuits with a wide variety of exercises have been developed. The training circuits are designed to be specific to the five training phases, which range from the novice to the advanced client.
 4. Repetition Ranges- Repetition will vary and be specific to the training phases, ranging from 6-25.

Training Techniques & Principles
How to Manipulate a Diet

As an individual gets in better shape, there will be times when results can slow down or even stop.

Temporarily shocking the body through diet manipulation is an excellent way to wake up a sluggish metabolism. Increasing or decreasing calories should be done only at certain times and not as the mainstay of a nutritional program. Increasing or decreasing calories should be done no longer than 1-3 weeks at a time.
This is a great technique, but it should be used sparingly.

Acceleration & Deceleration

Acceleration and deceleration are techniques that can be used in resistance training, cardio, and nutrition, the only three training areas that need to be manipulated when getting into shape. Acceleration and deceleration are excellent techniques, in any one of the three training areas, to shock the body for a temporary period of time. Sometimes through the course of training and nutrition, especially as an individual is getting closer to top shape, it will be more difficult to get the body to respond to resistance training, cardio, and nutrition.

Acceleration and deceleration can be applied simultaneously in the three training areas, as well as, applying them in only one or two of them. It depends on what the individual needs.

Acceleration and deceleration in the three training sessions are to help one get into shape. It's like driving a car. Sometimes you need to go fast (acceleration) and sometimes you need to put on the brakes (deceleration).

Combining Muscle Groups with Exercise

Exercising multiple muscle groups is a very efficient and effective way to train in a 30-minute resistance training session. An example of combining muscle groups follows: Body thru space lunge, stability ball hamstring kickbacks, triceps bench dips.

This combination of muscle group exercising is a way of training three different parts all at the same time (quads, hamstrings and triceps). This is an excellent way to thoroughly exhaust three different body parts all at once.

This is just an example of combining muscle groups in exercise. You can be as creative as you want in terms of which muscle groups to combine.

Partials

Partials are another set extension technique used to manipulate regular exercises. Partials can be used prior to, during, or after any exercise being performed. Generally, when training any body part, a full-range of motion is used. Partials are an excellent way to manipulate a regular exercise in order to increase the intensity, which will thoroughly exhaust the muscle.

Body Thru Space

Body thru space is yet another set extension technique that can be used to manipulate regular exercises. *It* means using <u>body weight</u> to perform an exercise. This can be done without using any rubber bands, dumbbells, or any kind of weight training machines. One clear example is for the chest: Instead of doing a dumbbell bench press (which is <u>not</u> a body thru space technique), the individual would do push-ups.

An example of a *body thru space* technique for legs would be lunges, as opposed to leg extensions, which are not considered body thru space. The body thru space technique can be used before or after a regular exercise, or even between regular exercises. This technique helps exhaust any muscle group much more efficiently.

Modify on the Fly

One of the worst things that can stifle results from an exercise program is BOREDOM. This often comes from doing the same workout for too long a period.

An interesting fact to know is that the body will start adapting to any kind of routine in about 21 days. So staying on the same exercise routine for more than three weeks hampers one's results. Therefore, variety is key to keeping the body off guard and never letting the muscle groups get adjusted to any kind of set routine.

Variety keeps workouts fresh and assures that results come on a consistent basis, which is the main objective.

The beauty of MCT™ principles and techniques is that the training applications are flexible, so people can modify their workouts whenever needed.

Life of a Rep

The life of a rep has to do with the quality of a set. It is not good enough to just do a bunch of reps during a set. The quality of the rep is extremely important. For example, if a set of 10 reps has been done, but only four of those were done properly, then 60% of that set was not performed to its highest potential.

The goal is to make sure every rep of every set counts, which means that every repetition being performed must be done with maximum efficiency. It's the quality – not quantity – that matters when performing reps for any body part.

Full vs. Partials

The purpose of doing an exercise through a full-range of motion is to thoroughly exhaust it from where it attaches at its origination and insertion points. Another benefit of a full-range exercise is that it promotes flexibility. However, only doing full-range motions, DOES NOT always thoroughly exhaust a muscle to its maximum potential. This is due to the fact that when a muscle is getting somewhat fatigued during a set, the tendency of momentum taking over or even stopping for a few seconds to rest before continuing the set allows the muscle just enough time to rest and not be trained properly.

This is when doing partial repetitions can be

applied, not only in the beginning of a full-range exercise as a pre-exhaust technique, but also in the middle of a set, as well as at the end.

Individuals should use full-range exercises as a foundation for training and use partials as their secret weapon to thoroughly exhaust all muscle groups.

Training Styles

There are three exercise training styles, which can be applied in the same workout session or in various combinations.

The three training styles are:
<u>Strict</u> Style Training
<u>Loose</u> Style Training
<u>Partial</u> Style Training

Strict style training can be used in various stages of any exercise program. It can be used whether the individual is a novice or advanced. Strict style training means keeping the exercise form strict and doing a full range of motion – with the exercise tempo being at a moderate speed. Strict training is excellent for developing a foundation for the novice who needs to learn how to perform exercises correctly, as well as for isolating a specific body part so that only that body part is being stimulated, without the assistance of other muscle groups.

Loose style training utilizes a full range of motion during each exercise. However, because it's used when lifting stronger resistance, the rep tempo is more upbeat and aggressive. Also, momentum and other muscle groups assist in the exercise of the specific body part being trained – but not at the expense of being out of control.

Partial style training can be applied anywhere during a set, and at any phase in training. Partials can be used in the beginning of a set as a pre-exhaust technique, as well as in the middle of a set, or even at the end of a set as a finishing technique. Partial training is an excellent way to push the muscle further than by only doing full-range of motion exercises. Please note, however, that partial training should not be applied solely on its own.

Exercise Selection Menu

The exercise selection menu serves as a tool which can be used by the individual in case there is a necessity to change an exercise from the main exercise program due to not having the right piece of equipment, or perhaps the exercise which is to be performed for that particular body part can not be performed because the necessary equipment is being used by other members in a busy gym or health club atmosphere.

On the following page there is a list of alternative exercises broken down by the different muscle groups, which can be used in case a variation from the exercise program is needed. Any exercise which is chosen will be correct.

How to Select the Proper Weight
All exercises have a range of repetitions that are to be performed. In order to determine a starting point, choose a weight so that it is possible to complete the repetitions that fall within the repetition ranges. If the weight is too heavy or too light make the necessary adjustments with each set or training round which is performed.

egs	Back	Chest	Shoulders	Triceps	Biceps	Calves	Abs
uat	DB Lying Pull - Over	Flat-BB Bench Press	Stand/Seat BB Shoulder Press	Close-Grip Bench Press	Stand BB Curl	BTS Toe Raise (off a platform)	Ball Crunch/Wind-mills
dified nges	Bent-Bar Row	DB Bench Press	DB Side Lateral Raise	Bench Dips	Stand/Seat ALT DB Curl	Donkey Calf Raises	Bicycle Crunch/ Flutter Kicks
nges	One-Arm DB Row	DB Flies	DB Front Raise	Stand/Seat DB Tri Ext			Hanging Knee Raises/ Kneel Cable Crunch
ain uat		Incline BB Bench Press	Stand/Seat DB Press	DB Triceps Kick-back	Stand Cable Curl		Hanging Knee Raises/ Kneel Cable Crunch
air uat		DB Bench Press					
ff- gged ad - t		Push ups					

Definitions of Abbreviations of Exercise Selection Menu

Dumb Bell	DB
Latissimus Dorsi	Lat
BarBell	BB
Extension	Ext
Body Thru Space	BTS
Triceps	Tri
Abdominals	Abs
Alternating	Alt

aining Phases

Base Training-Weeks 1-2

 The beginning of MCT™ is called *base training.* There are three circuits to be performed each session. There are 3 exercise rounds performed in each circuit. All 3 exercise rounds must be performed in their entirety before moving on to the next circuit.

In order to eliminate all of the guess-work, predetermined workouts are listed in the particular order to be performed.

Repetition ranges are to be kept between 8-12 for each training round and circuit

Rest periods are taken as needed between each training round

Abdominals are performed at the end once all of the circuits are completed

Explanation for Abdominals and Implementation

There is some confusion about the purpose of why and how much abdominal work should be done. The truth is that abs are a core muscle group and are involved throughout a MCT™ workout. Because of this, abs do not need a lot of work,

and yet one common misconception is that doing a lot of abs w
flatten the stomach and even burn body fat. This is not true.
Actually if too much abdominal work is done, the abdominal are
will protrude; after all it is a muscle.

However, it is useful to do some ab work. At the end of each
MCT™ weight training session, there is abdominal work
performed, just the right amount of work in order to tone the
area.

Abdominals are to be done at the end of the resistance training
sessions. They will be performed as three supersets, which mea
doing one exercise and immediately going to the next (Ex. Bicyc
Crunch and immediately doing Flutter Kicks).

A superset is exercising the same muscle group implementing a
different exercise. A group of abdominal exercises have been lis
with repetition ranges for each, which can be used throughout
MCT™. There are other ab exercises that can be used; however
the ones listed will be sufficient and can be used throughout
MCT™.

raining Phases	Weeks	Repetitions
ase Training	1-2	8-12
ndurance Training	3-4	12-15
ase Training	5-6	8-12
ndurance Training	7-8	12-15
ase Training	9-10	8-12
ndurance Training	11-12	12-15

xplanation of Training Phases

here are two training phases (Base Training, Endurance Training) that st 12 weeks, with repetitions ranging from 8-15.

e Automatic Body Balance Training System has been designed in a way at progressively becomes more challenging, in part due to the order of ercise changing as the individual is transitioning through each week, as ell as, repetitions changing on a regular basis

Base Training
Week 1

There are 3 exercise rounds performed in each circuit. All 3 exercise rounds must be performed in their entirety before moving on to the next circuit.

Day 1

Circuit 1

	Exercise	Reps
1	BTS Standing Calf Raise	8-12
2	Chair Squat	8-12
3	Bench Push Up Body thru Space	8-12

Circuit 2

	Exercise	Reps
4	Standing Dumbbell Curl	8-12
5	Stick Good Mornings	8-12
6	DB Stand Side Lateral Raises	8-12

Circuit 3

	Exercise	Reps
7	DB Alternate Leg Lunge	8-12
8	Stability Ball Ankle Weight Kick Back (Hamstring)	8-12
9	DB One Arm Row	8-12

Abdominals

3 Supersets	
Bicycle Crunch	25
Flutter Kicks	25

Day 2

Circuit 1

	Exercise	Reps
1	DB Triceps Kick Back	8-12
2	Stand DB Front Shoulder Raises	8-12
3	Bench Lying DB Pullover	8-12

Circuit 2

	Exercise	Reps
4	Body Bar Squat	8-12
5	One Arm DB Row	8-12
6	Standing DB Curl	8-12

Circuit 3

	Exercise	Reps
7	Incline DB Chest Press	8-12
8	Body Bar Bent Row	8-12
9	DB Flies	8-12

Abdominals

3 Supersets	
Ball Crunch	15-20
Windmills	15-20

Day 3

Circuit 1

	Exercise	Reps
1	Bench Lying DB Pullover	8-1
2	Standing Body Bar Upright Row	8-1
3	Side to Side Alternate Lunges	8-1

Circuit 2

	Exercise	Reps
4	Body Thru Space Platform Toe Raise	8-1
5	Alternating Seated DB Shoulder Press	8-1
6	Cambered Bar Slight Bent Knee Dead Lift	8-1

Circuit 3

	Exercise	Reps
7	Standing DB Hammer Curl	8-1
8	Curl Lunge (One Side at a Time)	8-1
9	Bench Push Ups (Body thru Space)	8-1

Abdominals

3 Supersets	
Hanging Knee Raises	20
Kneel Cable Crunch	20

Base Training
Week 2

ere are 3 exercise rounds performed in each circuit. All 3 exercise rounds must be
formed in their entirety before moving on to the next circuit.

Day 1

Circuit 1	
Exercise	Reps
Rubber Band Side Lunge Squat	8-12
Incline DB Chest Press	8-12
Seated DB Triceps Extension	8-12

Circuit 2	
Stick Good Mornings	8-12
Side Lateral Raises	8-12
Seated DB Curl	8-12

Circuit 3	
Body Bar DeadLift	8-12
Body Bar Bent Row	8-12
One Legged Platform BTS Toe Raise	8-12

Abdominals	
Supersets	
Cycle Crunch	25
Flutter Kicks	25

Day 2

Circuit 1	Exercise	Reps
1	DB Front Shoulder Raises	8-12
2	Lying DB Pullover	8-12
3	DB Triceps Kickback	8-12

Circuit 2	Exercise	Reps
4	One Arm DB Row	8-12
5	Standing DB Curl	8-12
6	Lunge Body Thru Space	8-12

Circuit 3	Exercise	Reps
7	Lying DB Pullover	8-12
8	Flat DB Flies	8-12
9	Incline DB Chest Press	8-12

Abdominals		
3 Supersets		
Ball Crunch		15-20
Windmills		15-20

Day 3

Circuit 1	Exercise	Reps
1	Stand Body Bar Upright Row	8-12
2	DB Squat	8-12
3	Body Bar Bent Row	8-12

Circuit 2	Exercise	Reps
4	Alternating Seated DB Shoulder Press	8-12
5	Deadlift	8-12
6	Donkey Calf Raises (Ankle Weights)	8-12

Circuit 3	Exercise	Reps
7	DB Squats	8-12
8	Bench Push Ups (Body Through Space)	8-12
9	Standing DB Curl	8-12

Abdominals		
3 Supersets		
Hanging Knee Raises		20
Kneel Cable Crunch		20

Training Phases

Endurance-Weeks 3-4

 The second training phase of MCT™ is called *endurance training.* Ther
are three circuits to be performed each session. There are 3 training
rounds performed in each circuit. All three training rounds must be
performed in their entirety before moving on to the next circuit.

In order to eliminate all of the guess-work, predetermined workouts ar
listed in the particular order to be performed.

Repetition ranges are to be kept between 12-15 for each training round
and circuit

Rest periods are taken as needed between each training round

Abdominals are performed at the end once all of the circuits are
completed

Endurance Training
Week 3

...e are 3 exercise rounds performed in each circuit. All 3 exercise rounds must be ...ormed in their entirety before moving on to the next circuit.

Day 1

Circuit 1	
...xercise	Reps
...B Curl Squats	12-15
...B Flat Bench Press	12-15
...onkey Calf Raise (...nkle Weights)	12-15

Circuit 2	
...B One Arm Row	12-15
...B Seated Shoulder ...ress	12-15
...B Seated Curl	12-15

Circuit 3	
...tanding Rubber ...and Kickbacks	12-15
...cline DB Flyes	12-15
...B Triceps ...ickback	12-15

Abdominals	
...ersets	
...le Crunch	25
...r Kicks	25

Day 2

Circuit 1		Exercise	Reps
	1	Rubber Band Slide Squat	12-15
	2	BTS Bench Pushups	12-15
	3	Bench Triceps Dips	12-15

Circuit 2			
	4	Lying DB Pullover	12-15
	5	Body Bar Front Shoulder Raise	12-15
	6	Stand Rubber Band Curl	12-15

Circuit 3			
	7	Wide Stance Straddle DB Squat	12-15
	8	Seated DB Triceps Extension	12-15
	9	Flat Close Grip Body Bar Bench Press	12-15

Abdominals			
3 Supersets			
Ball Crunch			15-20
Windmills			15-20

Day 3

Circuit 1		Exercise	Reps
	1	Body Thru Space One Legged Toe Raise	12-15
	2	Incline DB Flyes	12-15
	3	Bench Dip	12-15

Circuit 2			
	4	DB One Arm Row	12-15
	5	Side Lateral Raises	12-15
	6	Stand Body Bar Upright Row	12-15

Circuit 3			
	7	Rubber Band Side Step Squats	12-15
	8	Bench Push Ups	12-15
	9	DB Flat Bench	12-15

Abdominals			
3 Supersets			
Hanging Knee Raises			20
Kneel Cable Crunch			20

Endurance Training
Week 4

There are 3 exercise rounds performed in each circuit. All 3 exercise rounds must be performed in their entirety before moving on to the next circuit.

Day 1

Circuit 1

	Exercise	Reps
1	Body Bar Flat Bench Press	12-15
2	DB Flat Flyes	12-15
3	Donkey Calf Raise	12-15

Circuit 2

	Exercise	Reps
4	Body Bar Seat Shoulder Press	12-15
5	Body Bar Stand Curl	12-15
6	Seated DB Hammer Curl	12-15

Circuit 3

	Exercise	Reps
7	Incline DB Chest Press	12-15
8	Bench Pushups	12-15
9	Seated DB Triceps Extension	12-15

Abdominals

3 Supersets	
Bicycle Crunch	25
Flutter Kicks	25

Day 2

Circuit 1

	Exercise	Reps
1	Incline DB Flyes	12-15
2	DB Tri Kickback	12-15
3	Side To Side Leg Lunge	12-15

Circuit 2

	Exercise	Reps
4	DB Front Raise	12-15
5	Seated DB Curl	12-15
6	Bench DB Lying Pullover	12-15

Circuit 3

	Exercise	Reps
7	Incline Body Bar Chest Press	12-15
8	Triceps Kickbacks	12-15
9	DB Alternating Lunges	12-15

Abdominals

3 Supersets	
Ball Crunch	15-20
Windmills	15-20

Day 3

Circuit 1

	Exercise	Reps
1	Incline DB Chest Press	12-
2	Bench Triceps Dip	12-
3	Body Bar DeadLift	12-

Circuit 2

	Exercise	Reps
4	DB Side Lateral Raises	12-
5	Body Thru Space Platform Toe Raise	12-
6	Standing Stick Good Mornings	12-

Circuit 3

	Exercise	Reps
7	Bench Push Ups	12-
8	DB Flat Bench	12-
9	DB Triceps Kick Backs	12-

Abdominals

3 Supersets	
Hanging Knee Raises	20
Kneel Cable Crunch	20

Training Phases

Base Training-Weeks 5-6

The third training phase of MCT™ is called *base training.* There are three circuits to be performed each session. There are 3 training rounds performed in each circuit. All three training rounds must be performed in their entirety before moving on to the next circuit.

In order to eliminate all of the guess-work, the predetermined workouts have been listed in the particular order to be performed.

Repetition ranges are to be kept between 8-12 for each training round and circuit

Rest periods are taken as needed between each training round

Abdominals are performed at the end once all of the circuits are completed

Base Training
Week 5

There are 3 exercise rounds performed in each circuit. All 3 exercise rounds must be performed in their entirety before moving on to the next circuit.

Day 1		
Circuit 1		
	Exercise	Reps
1	DB Alternate Leg Lunge	8-12
2	Stability Ball Ankle Weight Kick Back (Hamstring)	8-12
3	DB One Arm Row	8-12
Circuit 2		
4	Standing Dumbbell Curl	8-12
5	Stick Good Mornings	8-12
6	DB Stand Side Lateral Raises	8-12
Circuit 3		
7	BTS Standing Calf Raise	8-12
8	Chair Squat	8-12
9	Bench Push Up (Bar) Body thru Space	8-12
Abdominals		
3 Supersets		
Bicycle Crunch		25
Flutter Kicks		25

Day 2		
Circuit 1		
	Exercise	Reps
1	Incline DB Chest Press	8-12
2	Body Bar Bent Row	8-12
3	DB Flies	8-12
Circuit 2		
4	Body Bar Squat	8-12
5	One Arm DB Row	8-12
6	Standing DB Curl	8-12
Circuit 3		
7	DB Triceps Kickback	8-12
8	Stand DB Front Shoulder Raises	8-12
9	Bench Lying DB Pullover	8-12
Abdominals		
3 Supersets		
Ball Crunch		15-20
Windmills		15-20

Day 3		
Circuit 1		
	Exercise	Reps
1	Standing DB Hammer Curl	8-12
2	DB Curl Lunge (One Side At A Time)	8-12
3	Bench Push Ups (Body Thru Space)	8-12
Circuit 2		
4	Body Thru Space Platform Toe Raise	8-12
5	Alternating Seated DB Shoulder Press	8-12
6	Cambered Bar Slight Bent Knee Deadlift	8-12
Circuit 3		
7	Bench Lying DB Pullover	8-12
8	Standing Body Bar Upright Row	8-12
9	Side To Side Alternate Lunges	8-12
Abdominals		
3 Supersets		
Hanging Knee Raises		20
Kneel Cable Crunch		20

Base Training
Week 6

There are 3 exercise rounds performed in each circuit. All 3 exercise rounds must be performed in their entirety before moving on to the next circuit.

Day 1

Circuit 1

	Exercise	Reps
	Body Bar DeadLift	8-12
	Body Bar Bent Row	8-12
	One Legged Platform BTS Toe Raise	8-12

Circuit 2

	Exercise	Reps
	Stick Good Mornings	8-12
	Side Lateral Raises	8-12
	Seated DB Curl	8-12

Circuit 3

	Exercise	Reps
	Rubber Band Side Lunge Squat	8-12
	Incline DB Chest Press	8-12
	Seated DB Triceps Extension	8-12

Abdominals

3 Supersets	
Cycle Crunch	25
Flutter Kicks	25

Day 2

Circuit 1

	Exercise	Reps
1	Lying DB Pullover	8-12
2	Flat DB Flies	8-12
3	Incline DB Chest Press	8-12

Circuit 2

	Exercise	Reps
4	One Arm DB Row	8-12
5	Standing DB Curl	8-12
6	Lunge Body Thru Space	8-12

Circuit 3

	Exercise	Reps
7	DB Front Shoulder Raises	8-12
8	Lying DB Pullover	8-12
9	DB Triceps Kickback	8-12

Abdominals

3 Supersets	
Ball Crunch	15-20
Windmills	15-20

Day 3

Circuit 1

	Exercise	Reps
1	DB Squats	8-12
2	Bench Push Ups (Body Thru Space)	8-12
3	Standing DB Curl	8-12

Circuit 2

	Exercise	Reps
4	Alternating Seated DB Shoulder Press	8-12
5	Deadlift	8-12
6	Donkey Calf Raises (Ankle Weights)	8-12

Circuit 3

	Exercise	Reps
7	Stand Body Bar Upright Row	8-12
8	DB Squat	8-12
9	Body Bar Bent Row	8-12

Abdominals

3 Supersets	
Hanging Knee Raises	20
Kneel Cable Crunch	20

Training Phases

Endurance Training-Weeks 7-8

 The fourth training phase of MCT™ is called *endurance training.* There are three circuits to be performed each session. There are 3 training rounds performed in each circuit. All three training rounds must be performed in their entirety before moving on to the next circuit.

In order to eliminate all of the guess-work, the predetermined workout have been listed in the particular order to be performed.

Repetition ranges are to be kept between 12-15 for each training round and circuit

Rest periods are taken as needed between each training round

Abdominals are performed at the end once all of the circuits are completed.

Endurance Training
Week 7

There are 3 exercise rounds performed in each circuit. All 3 exercise rounds must be performed in their entirety before moving on to the next circuit.

Day 1			Day 2			Day 3		
Circuit 1			**Circuit 1**			**Circuit 1**		
Exercise	Reps			Exercise	Reps			Exercise	Reps
Standing Rubber Band Kickbacks	12-15		1	Wide Stance Straddle DB Squat	12-15		1	Rubber Band Side Step Squats	12-15
Incline DB Flyes	12-15		2	Seated DB Triceps Extension	12-15		2	Bench Push Ups	12-15
DB Triceps Kickback	12-15		3	Flat Close Grip Body Bar Bench Press	12-15		3	DB Flat Bench	12-15
Circuit 2			**Circuit 2**			**Circuit 2**		
DB One Arm Row	12-15		4	Lying DB Pullover	12-15		4	DB One Arm Row	12-15
DB Seated Shoulder Press	12-15		5	Body Bar Front Shoulder Raise	12-15		5	Side Lateral Raises	12-15
Standing Rubber Band Kickbacks	12-15		6	Stand Rubber Band Curl	12-15		6	Stand Body Bar Upright Row	12-15
Circuit 3			**Circuit 3**			**Circuit 3**		
DB Curl Squats	12-15		7	Rubber Band Slide Squat	12-15		7	Body Thru Space One Legged Toe Raise	12-15
DB Flat Bench Press	12-15		8	BTS Bench Pushups	12-15		8	Incline DB Flyes	12-15
Donkey Calf Raise (Ankle Weights)	12-15		9	Bench Triceps Dips	12-15		9	Bench Dip	12-15
Abdominals			**Abdominals**			**Abdominals**		
Supersets			3 Supersets			3 Supersets		
Bicycle Crunch	25		Ball Crunch	15-20		Hanging Knee Raises	20
Flutter Kicks	25		Windmills	15-20		Kneel Cable Crunch	20

Endurance Training
Week 8

There are 3 exercise rounds performed in each circuit. All 3 exercise rounds must be performed in their entirety before moving on to the next circuit.

Day 1

Circuit 1

	Exercise	Reps
1	Incline DB Chest Press	12-15
2	Bench Pushups	12-15
3	Seated DB Triceps Extension	12-15

Circuit 2

4	Body Bar Seat Shoulder Press	12-15
5	Body Bar Stand Curl	12-15
6	Seated DB Hammer Curl	12-15

Circuit 3

7	Body Bar Flat Bench Press	12-15
8	DB Flat Flyes	12-15
9	Donkey Calf Raise	12-15

Abdominals

3 Supersets	
Bicycle Crunch	25
Flutter Kicks	25

Day 2

Circuit 1

	Exercise	Reps
1	Incline Body Bar Chest Press	12-15
2	Triceps Kickbacks	12-15
3	DB Alternating Lunges	12-15

Circuit 2

4	DB Front Raise	12-15
5	Seated DB Curl	12-15
6	Bench DB Lying Pullover	12-15

Circuit 3

7	Incline DB Flyes	12-15
8	DB Tri Kickback	12-15
9	Side To Side Leg Lunge	12-15

Abdominals

3 Supersets	
Ball Crunch	15-20
Windmills	15-20

Day 3

Circuit 1

	Exercise	Re...
1	Bench Push Ups	12
2	Bench Push Ups	12
3	DB Triceps Kick Backs	12

Circuit 2

4	DB Side Lateral Raises	12
5	Body Thru Space Platform Toe Raise	12
6	Standing Stick Good Mornings	12

Circuit 3

7	Incline DB Chest Press	12
8	Bench Triceps Dip	12
9	Body Bar DeadLift	12

Abdominals

3 Supersets	
Hanging Knee Raises	2(
Kneel Cable Crunch	2(

Training Phases

Base Training-Weeks 9-10

The fifth training phase of MCT™ is called *base training.* There are three circuits to be performed each session. There are 3 training rounds performed in each circuit. All three training rounds must be performed in their entirety before moving on to the next circuit.

In order to eliminate all of the guess-work predetermined workouts have been listed in the particular order to be performed.

Repetition ranges are to be kept between 8-12 for each training round and circuit

Rest periods are taken as needed between each training round

Abdominals are performed at the end once all of the circuits are completed

Base Training
Week 9

There are 3 exercise rounds performed in each circuit. All 3 exercise rounds must be performed in their entirety before moving on to the next circuit.

Day 1

	Exercise	Reps
	Circuit 1	
1	BTS Standing Calf Raise	8-12
2	Chair Squat	8-12
3	Bench Push Up (Bar) Body thru space	8-12
	Circuit 2	
4	Standing Dumbbell Curl	8-12
5	Stick Good Mornings	8-12
6	DB Stand Side Lateral Raises	8-12
	Circuit 3	
7	DB Alternate Leg Lunge	8-12
8	Stability Ball Ankle Weight Kick Back (Hamstring)	8-12
9	DB One Arm Row	8-12
	Abdominals	
	3 Supersets	
	Bicycle Crunch	25
	Flutter Kicks	25

Day 2

	Exercise	Reps
	Circuit 1	
1	DB Triceps Kickback	8-12
2	DB Triceps Kickback	8-12
3	Bench Lying DB Pullover	8-12
	Circuit 2	
4	Body Bar Squat	8-12
5	One Arm DB Row	8-12
6	Standing DB Curl	8-12
	Circuit 3	
7	Incline DB Chest Press	8-12
8	Body Bar Bent Row	8-12
9	DB Flies	8-12
	Abdominals	
	3 Supersets	
	Ball Crunch	15-20
	Windmills	15-20

Day 3

	Exercise	Rep
	Circuit 1	
1	Bench Lying DB Pullover	8-1
2	Standing Body Bar Upright Row	8-1
3	Side To Side Alternate Lunges	8-1
	Circuit 2	
4	Body Thru Space Platform Toe Raise	8-1
5	Alternating Seated DB Shoulder Press	8-1
6	Cambered Bar Slight Bent Knee Deadlift	8-1
	Circuit 3	
7	Standing DB Hammer Curl	8-1
8	DB Curl Lunge (One Side At A Time)	8-1
9	Bench Push Ups (Body Thru Space)	8-1
	Abdominals	
	3 Supersets	
	Hanging Knee Raises	20
	Kneel Cable Crunch	20

Base Training
Week 10

There are 3 exercise rounds performed in each circuit. All 3 exercise rounds must be performed in their entirety before moving on to the next circuit.

Day 1

Circuit 1

	Exercise	Reps
	Rubber Band Side Lunge Squat	8-12
	Incline DB Chest Press	8-12
	Seated DB Triceps Extension	8-12

Circuit 2

	Exercise	Reps
	Stick Good Mornings	8-12
	Side Lateral Raises	8-12
	Seated DB Curl	8-12

Circuit 3

	Exercise	Reps
	Body Bar DeadLift	8-12
	Body Bar Bent Row	8-12
	One Legged Platform BTS Toe Raise	8-12

Abdominals

Supersets	
Bicycle Crunch	25
Flutter Kicks	25

Day 2

Circuit 1

	Exercise	Reps
1	DB Front Shoulder Raises	8-12
2	DB Front Shoulder Raises	8-12
3	DB Triceps Kickback	8-12

Circuit 2

	Exercise	Reps
4	One Arm DB Row	8-12
5	Standing DB Curl	8-12
6	Lunge Body Thru Space	8-12

Circuit 3

	Exercise	Reps
7	Lying DB Pullover	8-12
8	Flat DB Flies	8-12
9	Incline DB Chest Press	8-12

Abdominals

3 Supersets	
Ball Crunch	15-20
Windmills	15-20

Day 3

Circuit 1

	Exercise	Reps
1	Stand Body Bar Upright Row	8-12
2	DB Squat	8-12
3	Body Bar Bent Row	8-12

Circuit 2

	Exercise	Reps
4	Alternating Seated DB Shoulder Press	8-12
5	Deadlift	8-12
6	Donkey Calf Raises (Ankle Weights)	8-12

Circuit 3

	Exercise	Reps
7	DB Squats	8-12
8	Bench Push Ups (Body Thru Space)	8-12
9	Standing DB Curl	8-12

Abdominals

3 Supersets	
Hanging Knee Raises	20
Kneel Cable Crunch	20

Training Phases

Endurance Training-Weeks 11-12

The fourth training phase of MCT™ is called *endurance training.* There are three circuits to be performed each session. There are 3 training rounds performed in each circuit. All three training rounds must be performed in their entirety before moving on to the next circuit.

In order to eliminate all of the guess-work, predetermined workouts have been listed in the particular order to be performed.

Repetition ranges are to be kept between 12-15 for each training round and circuit

Rest periods are taken as needed between each training round

Abdominals are performed at the end once all of the circuits are completed.

Endurance Training
Week 11

There are 3 exercise rounds performed in each circuit. All 3 exercise rounds must be performed in their entirety before moving on to the next circuit.

Day 1

Circuit 1	
Exercise	Reps
DB One Arm Row	12-15
DB Seated Shoulder Press	12-15
DB Seated Curl	12-15

Circuit 2	
DB Curl Squats	12-15
DB Flat Bench Press	12-15
Donkey Calf Raise (Ankle Weights)	12-15

Circuit 3	
Standing Rubber Band Kickbacks	12-15
Incline DB Flyes	12-15
Incline DB Flies	12-15

Abdominals	
3 Supersets	
Bicycle Crunch	25
Flutter Kicks	25

Day 2

Circuit 1		
	Exercise	Reps
1	Lying DB Pullover	12-15
2	Body Bar Front Shoulder Raise	12-15
3	Stand Rubber Band Curl	12-15

Circuit 2		
4	Rubber Band Slide Squat	12-15
5	BTS Bench Pushups	12-15
6	Bench Triceps Dips	12-15

Circuit 3		
7	Wide Stance Straddle DB Squat	12-15
8	Seated DB Triceps Extension	12-15
9	Flat Close Grip Body Bar Bench Press	12-15

Abdominals		
3 Supersets		
Ball Crunch		15-20
Windmills		15-20

Day 3

Circuit 1		
	Exercise	Reps
1	DB One Arm Row	12-15
2	Side Lateral Raises	12-15
3	Stand Body Bar Upright Row	12-15

Circuit 2		
4	Body Thru Space One Legged Toe Raise	12-15
5	Incline DB Flyes	12-15
6	Bench Dip	12-15

Circuit 3		
7	Rubber Band Side Step Squats	12-15
8	Bench Push Ups	12-15
9	DB Flat Bench	12-15

Abdominals		
3 Supersets		
Hanging Knee Raises		20
Kneel Cable Crunch		20

Endurance Training
Week 12

There are 3 exercise rounds performed in each circuit. All 3 exercise rounds must be performed in their entirety before moving on to the next circuit.

Day 1		
Circuit 1		
	Exercise	Reps
1	Body Bar Seat Shoulder Press	12-15
2	Body Bar Stand Curl	12-15
3	Seated DB Hammer Curl	12-15
Circuit 2		
4	Body Bar Flat Bench Press	12-15
5	DB Flat Flyes	12-15
6	Donkey Calf Raise	12-15
Circuit 3		
7	Incline DB Chest Press	12-15
8	Bench Pushups	12-15
9	Seated DB Triceps Extension	12-15
Abdominals		
3 Supersets		
Bicycle Crunch		25
Flutter Kicks		25

Day 2		
Circuit 1		
	Exercise	Reps
1	DB Front Raise	12-15
2	Seated DB Curl	12-15
3	Bench DB Lying Pullover	12-15
Circuit 2		
4	Incline DB Flyes	12-15
5	Seated DB Raise	12-15
6	Side To Side Leg Lunge	12-15
Circuit 3		
7	Incline Body Bar Chest Press	12-15
8	Triceps Kickbacks	12-15
9	DB Alternating Lunges	12-15
Abdominals		
3 Supersets		
Ball Crunch		15-20
Windmills		15-20

Day 3		
Circuit 1		
	Exercise	Reps
1	DB Side Lateral Raises	12-15
2	Body Thru Space Platform Toe Raise	12-15
3	Standing Stick Good Mornings	12-15
Circuit 2		
4	Incline DB Chest Press	12-15
5	Bench Triceps Dip	12-15
6	Body Bar DeadLift	12-15
Circuit 3		
7	Bench Push Ups	12-15
8	DB Flat Bench	12-15
9	DB Triceps Kick Backs	12-15
Abdominals		
3 Supersets		
Hanging Knee Raises		20
Kneel Cable Crunch		20

Congratulations

You have completed the 12 week Automatic Body Balance program. The next step is to repeat again and start at week 1.

Enjoy the new stronger you!